CATEGORY: OPTHALMc

DRS BRAY, SMITH,
TANNA & WHITER
St. Andrews Medical
50 Oakleigh Road Nc
Whetstone London N
Tel: 020 8445 0475

GU01218270

Seasonal allergic conjunctivitis and rhinoconjunctivitis

Edited by

David Easty and Richard Wyse

Proceedings of a Round Table discussion held at
the Royal Society of Medicine, London, UK, on
19 December 2002. These discussions reflect the
experience and opinions of the panellists and do
not necessarily reflect the opinions of the Royal
Society of Medicine nor the recommendations of
Alcon Laboratories.

*Published by the Royal Society of Medicine Press
Limited with financial support from Alcon
Laboratories.*

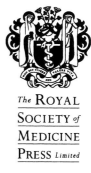

The ROYAL
SOCIETY *of*
MEDICINE
PRESS *Limited*

©2003 Royal Society of Medicine Press Limited
1 Wimpole Street, London W1G 0AE, UK
www.rsmpress.ac.uk

Customers in North America should order via:
RSM Press, c/o Jamco Distribution Inc., 1401 Lakeway Drive,
Lewisville, TX 75057, USA. Tel: +1 800 538 1287 (toll free); Fax: +1 972 353 1303.
Email: jamco@majors.com

These proceedings are published by the Royal Society of Medicine
Press Ltd with financial support from the sponsor. The contributors
are responsible for the scientific content and for the views expressed,
which are not necessarily those of the sponsor, of the editor of the
series or of the volume, of the Royal Society of Medicine or of the
Royal Society of Medicine Press Ltd. Distribution has been in
accordance with the wishes of the sponsor but a copy is available to
any fellow of the Society at a privileged price.

British Library Cataloguing in Publication Data
A catalogue record for this book is available from the British Library

ISBN 1-85315-554-3
ISSN 0268-3091

Phototypeset by Phoenix Photosetting, Chatham, Kent
Printed in Great Britain by Ebenezer Baylis, The Trinity Press, Worcester

Participants

CHAIRMAN
Professor David Easty, MD, FRCS, FRC Ophth
Emeritus Professor of Ophthalmology, Department of Ophthalmology, University of Bristol, at Bristol Eye Hospital, Lower Maudlin Street, Bristol, UK

PARTICIPANTS
Professor Mark Abelson, MD, CM, FRCS(C)
Associate Clinical Professor, Harvard Medical School, Boston, MA, USA; Senior Clinical Scientist, Schepens Eye Research Institute, Boston, MA, USA; Advisory Board, Faculty of Medicine, McGill University, Montreal, Quebec, Canada; Ophthalmic Research Associates, Inc., North Andover, MA, USA

Professor Martin Church, M Pharm, PhD, DSc
Division of Infection, Inflammation and Repair, School of Medicine, University of Southampton, Southampton, UK

Mr James McGill, MA, D Phil, FRCS, FRC Ophth
Southampton Eye Unit, Southampton General Hospital, Tremona Road, Southampton, UK

Dr Dermot Ryan, MB BCh, BAO, MRCGP, MICGP, DCH, D Obst RCPI
General Practitioner, Woodbrook Medical Centre, Loughborough, UK
and Clinical Research Fellow (Primary care respiratory medicine), University of Aberdeen, UK

Dr Richard Wyse, FRSM
Medical Director, Celsius Ltd, London, UK; Department of Surgery, Hammersmith Hospital, London, UK

Contents

Seasonal allergic conjunctivitis
David Easty

The field of seasonal allergic conjunctivitis has produced a surprisingly vast amount of literature. The participants at this meeting came together to discuss the basic science, clinical situation and treatment options with respect to general practice.

Examination of the eye

It is important that general practitioners, whenever possible, perform a basic but thorough examination of the eye in their patients. When visual acuity is not assessed, undiagnosed eye disease will be overlooked. For example, patients with diabetes mellitus can develop ocular complications that lead to sight loss (even those with insulin-dependent diabetes). It is up to the general practitioner to identify eye disease, from whatever cause, using a few simple examination methods.

Distance visual acuity can be determined using the standard Snellen test chart, followed by the use of the pinhole test, which involves looking at the test chart through a pinhole disc. When the patient has reduced distance vision due to a refractive error, such as short-sightedness, this test will improve the visual acuity to almost normal levels (6/6). When the vision is not improved there may be a disease present, such as cataract or involutional macular degeneration.

General practitioners need only very simple equipment and materials to carry out a satisfactory examination, such as a small magnifier, an ophthalmoscope, topical eye drops containing anaesthetic, a short-acting mydriatic (tropicamide) and some fluorescein. The ophthalmoscope is used to examine the anterior segment (with a +12DS lens in the eye piece), as well as the retina and the optic disc.

Figure 1 shows the anatomy of the anterior segment of the eye and highlights the simple structure of the tarsal, bulbar conjunctiva and fornices. Other structures of the eye include the lashes, ducts and Meibomian glands. The important function of the structures of the external eye is to protect the integrity and clarity of the cornea, which is the main focussing lens of the eye. The external eye should be examined to check the cornea for transparency and foreign bodies. A fluorescein drop will highlight damage to the corneal epithelium, such as a traumatic abrasion, or a dendritic ulcer due to herpes simplex virus. The bulbar conjunctiva should be examined in different positions of gaze, and the upper and lower tarsal plates should be everted. The preauricular lymph nodes may be palpable in certain infections, eg in adenovirus conjunctivitis.

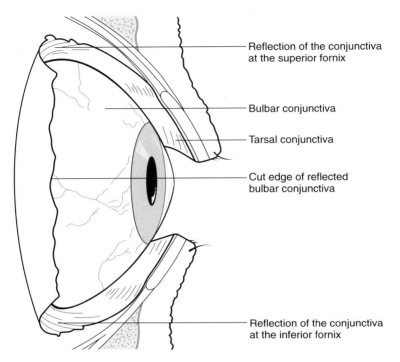

FIGURE I The conjunctival sac, lining the sclera (bulbar conjunctiva) and the tarsal plates. The upper and lower cul-de-sacs are known as the fornices

Reproduced with permission from Ragge NK, Easty DL. *Immediate eye care: an illustrated manual.* St Louis: Mosby International, 1990

Examination of the posterior segment with an ophthalmoscope can reveal several quite common diseases, including of course a cataract, but also macular degeneration and chronic simple glaucoma.

Chronic simple glaucoma, seen in elderly patients, involves an increasing degree of excavation or cupping of the optic disc. In glaucoma, the optic disc looks pale and, although cupping may not be obvious, a difference in the diameter of the cup on each side may mean that the patient should be referred to a hospital eye department.

Most people with seasonal allergic conjunctivitis are in the younger age group and they are unlikely to have cataract, macular disease or glaucoma. They may be diabetic, however, so the first visit of a patient with eye problems should include a retinal examination. A proper examination of the retina involves pupil dilation with tropicamide drops, which are short acting — only lasting for about two hours. (It must be remembered that the near vision is compromised during this time because of temporary loss of the accommodation.)

Conjunctivitis

Seasonal allergic conjunctivitis and perennial allergic conjunctivitis

Seasonal allergic conjunctivitis and perennial allergic conjunctivitis are the most common disorders of the eye, with seasonal allergic conjunctivitis the more common of the two [1]. It is often associated with allergic rhinitis, hence the term rhinoconjunctivitis used in the title of this publication. Seasonal and perennial allergic conjunctivitis are also the least severe eye disorders. Both are seen and managed more often in general practice than in hospital practice, although perennial allergic conjunctivitis is more likely to be managed in the hospital service because it is chronic and caused by a different kind of allergen.

Vernal keratoconjunctivitis

Vernal keratoconjunctivitis, which is severe, is seen in children from 5–15 years of age and lasts for 5–10 years. It is characterized by vernal catarrh, a severe allergy of the tarsal conjunctiva in children, which can lead to the development of corneal ulcers [2, 3]. It is characterized by large cobblestone papillae situated on the conjunctival surfaces of the upper tarsal plates. In very active cases, large amounts of thick mucus stick to the surface of the cornea, which can cause an ulcer and loss of vision. The conjunctiva at the edge of the cornea (limbus) becomes swollen, hyperaemic and infiltrated by foci of inflammatory cells. Vernal keratoconjunctivitis is different from seasonal and perennial allergic conjunctivitis because it is more severe and should be under the care of an ophthalmologist. It is associated with other atopic conditions: 60% of patients have eczema and 60% have asthma — only about 10–20% have no associated atopic condition. Antihistamines and mast cell stabilizers are inadequate, so topical steroids need to be given under specialist supervision, and the general practitioner should refer the patient to hospital when there is active inflammation.

Atopic conjunctivitis

Atopic conjunctivitis, or keratoconjunctivitis, occurs more often in older patients [1]; it is an adult form of allergic eye disease that, fortunately, is relatively rare. It usually appears at the age of 25–30 years. The large papilli and cobblestone appearance seen with vernal conjunctivitis are not seen in this condition; the papillae are small and diffuse, with many packed together tightly. The vertical blood vessels seen in the normal tarsal plate of a healthy patient are not visible in atopic conjunctivitis because they are hidden by the inflammation and papillae. The condition is caused by an allergic response and patients are highly atopic.

Giant papillary conjunctivitis

Giant papillary conjunctivitis is similar in appearance to atopic conjunctivitis. It is very rare and is usually seen in association with contact lens wear or in the presence of foreign objects in the conjunctival sac—for example, protruding sutures after a graft or cataract extraction. It is caused by a localized sensitivity to a rough or foreign body surface. It produces cobblestone papillae (3–4 mm in diameter) that are generally smaller and flatter than those seen in vernal keratoconjunctivitis.

Seasonal allergic conjunctivitis

Causes, signs and symptoms

The causes of allergic conjunctivitis are well known. Airborne allergens are mostly responsible for seasonal allergic conjunctivitis, including ragweed pollen, particularly in the USA, and grass, tree and weed pollens in the UK. Animal dander and house-dust mites are the usual causes of perennial allergic conjunctivitis.

The symptoms of seasonal allergic conjunctivitis include:

- itching
- soreness
- stinging
- watering.

Seasonal allergic conjunctivitis is a bilateral disease and is usually symmetrical. Chemosis (conjunctival oedema) may be observed and there also may be hyperaemia of the bulbar conjunctiva, watering and a small amount of mucin. Hyperaemia of the tarsal everted plates is characteristic, and the lids will be swollen. Perennial conjunctivitis occurs throughout the year and is due to a persistent environmental allergen.

Figure 2 shows the typical appearance of seasonal allergic conjunctivitis. A few papilliae are evident and the tarsal plate is almost normal. Signs are not present in the lower tarsal plate, but there is chemosis (swelling and oedema) of the conjunctiva. In most cases, seasonal allergic conjunctivitis is associated with allergic rhinitis.

Investigations and diagnosis

When a patient presents with symptoms in their eyes, investigations should include a full examination of the external eye, with cultures taken from the conjunctiva and

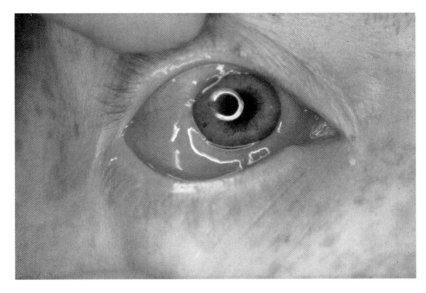

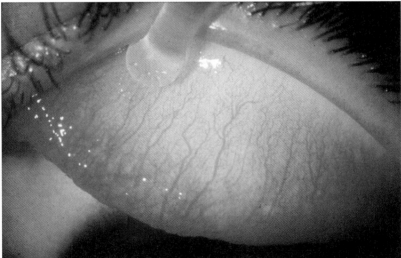

FIGURE 2   Appearance of seasonal allergic conjunctivitis

lid margins to eliminate the presence of infectious microorganisms. Skin prick tests may be useful. More specialist tests might include serum immunoglobulin (Ig) E (particularly in vernal keratoconjunctivitis) and the radioallergosorbent test (RAST), which gives an indication of the magnitude of the IgE response.

Although careful examination is essential, some signs may be absent because the condition is seasonal. History taking is important: complaints of itching are a very strong indicator of allergy and the symptoms will more often occur outdoors in seasonal allergic conjunctivitis and indoors in perennial allergic conjunctivitis.

Differential diagnosis

In the primary care situation, the doctor must be sure to exclude other forms of external eye disease. Table I shows the differential diagnoses for red eye. In a patient who presents with symptoms typical of allergy, the doctor should consider the following possibilities:

- keratoconjunctivitis sicca, in which the eyes are dry, sandy and gritty, and the symptoms are worse at the end of the day
- meibomitis, which is difficult to diagnose, in which the eyes feel sandy and gritty and probably feel worse in the morning
- anterior blepharitis, which presents with crusting and irritation of the lid margins
- medicamentosa: in which ocular medications cause conjunctivitis, particularly after delayed-type hypersensitivity problems; these affect the eye itself, as well as the skin in and around the treated eye
- lacrimal gland drainage obstruction.

TABLE I   Differential diagnoses for red eye and dry eye

Possible cause	Possible condition
Allergic	● Acute
	– seasonal
	– perennial
	● Chronic
	– vernal keratoconjunctivitis
	– atopic keratoconjunctivitis
	– giant papillary
Autoimmune	● Scleritis
	● Uveitis
Non-specific	● Dry eye (keratoconjunctivitis sicca)
	● Subtarsal foreign body
	● Blepharitis
	● Chemical toxicity

Dry eye must be kept in mind, although it would be difficult for the erosions that occur to be seen in general practice. Differential diagnoses include:

- nocturnal lagophthalmos (in which the eye does not always close at night), which results in drying and erosions on the surface because of the separation between the lids
- subtarsal foreign body, which could be revealed by examination of the underneath of the tarsal plate
- hypochondriasis, which can be time consuming because ultimately no diagnosis can be made.

Treatments

As a first step, the causative allergen should be identified, preferably by skin testing [4]. Once identified, the allergen — eg pet dander, feather-containing pillows, quilts and wool blankets — should be eliminated wherever possible. Positive changes to the environment, such as the introduction of air conditioning, can help when feasible. Desensitization is not used so commonly now because of rumours that it is dangerous [5]. In cases in which an antigen is causing an acute response in the eye, good results can be obtained by diluting the antigen, perhaps with tear substitutes.

Recommended topical treatments according to the British National Formulary, include some antihistamines active at H_1- and H_2-receptors and mast cell stabilizers:

- antazoline
- azelastine
- emedastine
- fluorometholone
- levocabastine
- lodoxamide
- nedocromil
- sodium cromoglycate.

Topical corticosteroids usually are not necessary in patients with seasonal allergic conjunctivitis and they should be used only under expert supervision, which should include a drug treatment letter and follow-up through the hospital's eye service [6]. Such precautions are necessary because these drugs might increase the frequency of recurrence of herpes simplex [3], and they do increase the intraocular pressure after long-term use in the eye [4]. Both systemic and topical steroids can cause cataracts.

Research considerations

Seasonal allergic conjunctivitis seems to fulfil Koch's postulates. One or more positive allergens may be found, a specific antibody has been identified, an animal model has been produced and adoptive transfer techniques can be used (the antibody can be transferred to another animal that is not sensitized to reproduce the disease process).

Two models are used in laboratory research: an active model of conjunctival immediate hypersensitivity and a passive model [7, 8]. The active model involves sensitization with ovalbumin and adjuvant. At 21 days, production of ovalbumin-specific IgE and IgG is observed. Challenge involves topical application of ovalbumin to one eye only. Degranulation of mast cells occurs for up to one hour and then stops (Figure 3). At four hours, no further mast cell degranulation occurs. This model can be used as a test system for new therapeutic compounds. However, it suffers from unpredictability at times.

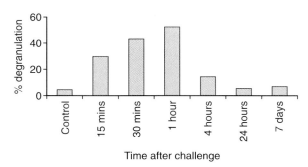

FIGURE 3 Percentage of degranulated mast cells from challenged tissue in an active model of seasonal allergic conjunctivitis

In the passive model, systemic specific antibody is introduced. Topical introduction of ovalbumin induces an immediate conjunctival allergic reaction/allergy. Figure 4 shows the dose–response of sodium cromoglycate and of nedocromil sodium tested in this model. Such animal models may be useful, as may the conjunctival challenge test.

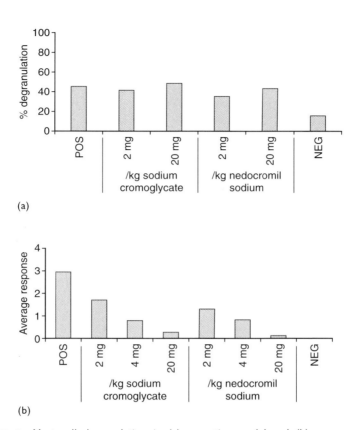

FIGURE 4 Mast cell degranulation in (a) an active model and (b) average clinical response in a passive model after application of drugs

Summary

This chapter concerns the main allergic diseases of the external eye, involving mast cell degranulation and immediate hypersensitivity. The meeting paid little attention to severe allergic conditions such as vernal keratoconjunctivitis or atopic conjunctivitis, but concentrated on seasonal rhinoconjunctivitis and perennial allergic conjunctivitis, both of which are common conditions likely to be diagnosed and treated by general practitioners. A large number of reputed treatments are available that will go some way to help the many patients that suffer from these conditions.

References

1. Bielory L. Allergic and immunologic disorders of the eye. Part II: ocular allergy. J Allergy Clin Immunol 2000; **106(6)**: 1019–32.

2. Fonacier L, Luchs J, Udell I. Ocular allergies. Curr Allergy Asthma Rep 2001; **1(4)**: 389–96.

3. Frankland AW, Easty D. Vernal kerato-conjunctivitis: an atopic disease. Trans Ophthalmol Soc UK 1971; **91**: 479–82.

4. Bremond-Gignac D, Beydon N, Laroche L. Skin tests and cutaneous allergy in children with ocular allergy. Acta Ophthalmol Scand Suppl 2000; **230**: 76–7.

5. Vourdas D, Syrigou E, Potamianou P, et al. Double-blind, placebo-controlled evaluation of sublingual immunotherapy with standardized olive pollen extract in pediatric patients with allergic rhinoconjunctivitis and mild asthma due to olive pollen sensitization. Allergy 1998; **53(7)**: 662–72.

6. Joss JD, Craig TJ. Seasonal allergic conjunctivitis: overview and treatment update. J Am Osteopath Assoc 1999; **99(Suppl 7)**: S13–18.

7. Doherty MJ, Easty DL. Inflammatory and immunological cell profiles in a rat model of conjunctival immediate hypersensitivity. Clin Exp Allergy 1989; **19(4)**: 449–55.

8. McGrath LE, Doherty MJ, Easty DL, Norris A. Nedocromil sodium in two models of conjunctival immediate hypersensitivity. Adv Ther 2000; **17(1)**: 7–13.

A primary care perspective

Dermot Ryan

In the UK, 90% of all patient contacts are provided in primary care, which receives approximately 25% of the total resource for health care [2]. The average general practitioner has a list size of 1800 personal patients, ranging from 400 in the Scottish islands up to about 3500 in inner city London, Leicester, Manchester and Birmingham [3]. General practitioners in the UK carry out approximately 250 million consultations per annum [4], however, they are grossly under-resourced and have limited facilities in terms of time, equipment and training. This makes a thorough examination of the eye, as espoused by ophthalmologists for consultations relating to eye problems, virtually impossible to provide. However, ocular examination in the elderly or symptomatic patients must be performed.

Secondary care accounts for most of the rest of patient contacts. In the UK, the average district general hospital provides population health services for 250,000–300,000 people. Secondary care services are agglomerating; for example, in Leicestershire, the University Hospitals of Leicester NHS Trust — which comprises three acute hospitals — provides secondary and tertiary care services for 950,000 patients. Tertiary care specialists are relatively uncommon in the UK, although they are rapidly increasing in numbers.

Allergy

Allergy is a systemic disorder that presents as an abnormal response to substances in the patient's environment. Allergy may manifest itself in the form of drug reactions, asthma, eczema, urticaria, food intolerance, rhinitis and conjunctivitis. In primary care, allergic conjunctivitis normally presents in combination with rhinitis, most frequently as hay fever. A recent Medline search with the headings 'allergic conjunctivitis' and the subheadings 'immunology, prevention and control, and epidemiology' found 174 citations. A search for 'conjunctivitis, allergy and primary care' found no citations: it would seem that currently no body of research exists on seasonal allergic conjunctivitis in primary care.

Prevalence

Allergic disease is increasing in prevalence throughout the developing world and it is also increasing in prevalence in African and Asian countries as they become more westernized and acquire carpets, central heating and refined food. The Isaac study found a prevalence of asthma alone of about 8%, but the prevalence was 20% when asthma was considered in combination with other allergic diseases — such as atopic dermatitis and allergic rhinoconjunctivitis (Figure 1) [5]. Allergic complaints are a very common reason for presentation to general practice. In the UK, 33% of children will have had a wheezing episode by the age of 12 years and 18% will have comp ained

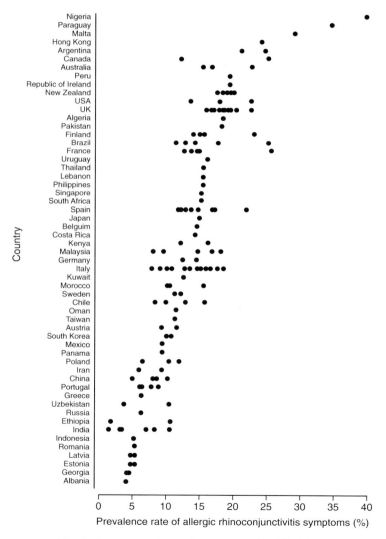

FIGURE 1   Allergic disease: prevalence of symptoms in 463,801 children aged 13–14 years. Adapted from Isaac, 1998 [5]

of rhinoconjunctivitis in the previous year, with a cumulative prevalence of over 35% [6]. Such episodes may not be 'true asthma', but they will encompass the asthma syndrome, as most wheezing in children aged under three years is virally induced rather than allergy based (although allergy-based asthma can start early). Most cases of allergic rhinoconjunctivitis are seen by general practitioners during the hay fever season, which lasts from approximately mid-April to the beginning of July in the UK.

Risk factors

The risk factors for allergy are well known:

- genetic predisposition
- exposure to allergens
- environmental factors.

Allergens are more prevalent than ever before, in part due to modem lifestyles that include air conditioning, central heating, carpets, increased hygiene, increased humidity in the home (which encourages the growth of house-dust mites) and pets inside the home. The hygiene hypothesis suggests that because our lives are sanitized, we are less exposed to infection and infestation than in the past. Previously the efforts of the immune system were employed in combating infection and infestation – in the absence of such infections, when our immune system encounters small amounts of foreign proteins, it mounts an attack manifesting as allergic disease. The external environment also contributes and impacts upon pre-existing allergic disease—although it is not recognized absolutely as a cause or factor in allergic disease, it definitely exacerbates allergy. For example, temperature inversion, low ground level ozone and high levels of PM10s (particulate air pollutants) during the hay fever season leads to an increase in both number of cases and severity of allergic rhinoconjunctivitis.

Good anti-allergy practice programme

The Good Anti-Allergy Practice Programme (GAAPP) studied management of allergy, particularly hay fever, in primary care [7]. A questionnaire was sent to 300 general practitioners to evaluate their knowledge and practice, to compare findings with the gold standard from the consensus statement on the treatment of allergic rhinitis [8] and to measure practice with four standards assessed through 21 criteria (Table 1). Table 1 shows results from the GAAPP study, which was presented at the 2001 scientific meeting of the British Society of Allergy and Clinical Immunology.

Results of this study suggest that general practitioners tend not to ask questions about symptoms. This is probably because patients tell their doctor what is wrong with them—they complain of itching, sneezing or a runny or blocked nose, or they

TABLE 1   National results of the GAAPP survey

Standard	Criterion		Number (%) of general practitioners meeting criterion
1	1	Itchy nose	32.6
	2	Sneezing	67.4
	3	Runny nose, rhinorrhea	90.5
	4	Blocked nose, nasal obstruction	65.7
2	5	Asks about allergies (family or personal)	92.7
	6	Asks about general medical history (family or personal)	91.6
	7	Asks about symptoms patients gets	42.7
	8	Asks about treatment patient has tried	56.2
3	9	Checks for asthma or breathing problems	44.4
	10	Checks for skin problems	9.6
	11	Checks for pollen-related food allergies	1.7
	12	Looks up patients nose (looking for physical obstruction)	91
	13	Does skin prick test	5.6
	14	Tests for immunoglobulin E or radioallergosorbent tests	11.8
4	15	Advise prevention of contact with allergic substance	14
	16	Identify and avoid allergen	39.9
	17	Remove allergen from patient's environment	12.4
	18	Mild seasonal allergic rhinitis treated with antihistamines if season started, cromones if not	97.2
	19	Moderate or uncontrolled mild seasonal allergic rhinitis treated with nasal steroid spray. Treat eyes with drops if necessary	92.7
	20	Severe or uncontrolled moderate seasonal allergic rhinitis, combine steroid nasal spray and antihistamine spray	37.1
	21	If still uncontrolled, add decongestant, ipatroprium bromide for the runny nose, pain killers if necessary or a short course of steroid tablets	8.4

actually may say they have hay fever. Most general practitioners do ask about allergies (92.7%) and review the patient's general medical history (91.6%). Some clarify the patients' symptoms and ask about treatments the patient has tried. In the UK, as in other countries, most treatments are available over the counter and the pharmacy is the first port of call, so most people will have tried at least one or two drugs before visiting their general practitioner.

The study suggests that general practitioners do not usually check for asthma or breathing problems, despite the association between allergic rhinitis and asthma. Skin problems and pollen-related food allergies usually are not discussed either — in general, doctors in the UK seem to have very little awareness of pollen-related food allergies. Most general practitioners examine the patient's nose, but few do skin prick, immunoglobulin E or radioallergosorbent tests because they are not available to most doctors. Doctors do try to identify the allergen where possible, but very few advise their patients to avoid contact with the allergic substance, because most patients have already recognized and avoided the allergen themselves — typically horses or pollens. Although studies show that removing the allergen from the patient's environment may give short-term relief, it is not a particularly useful strategy in the long term, particularly given people's reluctance to remove pets from their homes [8].

The GAAPP results show that 97.2% of general practitioners treat seasonal allergic rhinitis with antihistamines or cromones (cromoglycate and nedocromil) when the season has started. In addition, 92.7% of general practitioners treat mild or uncontrolled mild seasonal allergic rhinitis, including conjunctivitis, with nasal steroid sprays, and eye symptoms with drops, usually cromoglycate, nedocromil sodium or topical antihistamines. Overall, 50% of general practitioners aim to resolve their patients' eye problems. Patients should not need to be referred to hospital or an ophthalmologist because of an allergic eye condition; the main reasons for ophthalmic referral would be glaucoma, cataracts, resistant styes or cysts in the eyes, or acutely painful red eyes, the cause of which cannot be diagnosed in the surgery. A diagnosis of allergic conjunctivitis not responding to standard treatment would warrant referral.

Treatment approaches in general practice

Allergic rhinitis and its impact on asthma (ARIA) is a non-governmental organization that works in collaboration with the World Health Organization. Currently the ARIA guidelines are at the level of consensus, but as they evolve, they will review and incorporate research findings [9]. ARIA indicates that atopy is a systemic disease that encompasses:

- anaphylaxis
- rhinitis
- asthma

- conjunctivitis
- dermatitis
- urticaria.

Most general practitioners understand these relationships, but are not interested in the minutiae of the pathophysiology with the complex interactions of chemokines and cytokines, such as immunoglobulin E, adhesion molecules and interleukins, because they are not perceived as relevant to their day-to-day practice.

The British Society of Allergy and Clinical Immunology (BSACI) guidelines recommended a treatment pathway that starts with treating rhinitis with antihistamines and involves the addition of topical nasal steroids if control is not achieved (Figure 2) [10–12]. This reflects current practice in primary care. If neither class of agent works alone, a combination of topical steroids and antihistamines is generally used. Any and all of these options should be underpinned by guidance on allergen avoidance: eg not going out in the early evening, wearing sunglasses, and so on. The role of leukotriene receptor antagonists has not been fully established, but in some patients they can be very useful [13].

Immunotherapy may be suitable for selected patients with immunoglobulin E-mediated rhinitis and asthma. In practice, such therapy is not used in the primary care setting in the UK. This is because the Department of Health issued guidelines in 1985 stating that full resuscitation facilities must be available when administering such therapy. As a result, it is only given in specialist centres, of which there are very few in the UK [14]. Occasionally, referral for surgery is indicated for hypertrophy of the turbinates or deviation of the nasal septum.

The evidence on treatment of rhinitis in the ARIA guidelines shows that all treatments except allergen avoidance are useful for eye symptoms (Table 2). Antihistamines and intranasal steroids both have beneficial effects on eye symptoms, as do topical cromones. Nedocromil can be used twice a day, whereas sodium cromoglycate needs to be used many times a day — up to 10 times — in order to be effective. Evidence also shows that anti-leukotriene agents can control eye symptoms in patients with allergic rhinitis.

Gøtzsche and colleagues performed a meta-analysis of studies of house-dust mite avoidance [10]. This showed that allergen avoidance (specifically by measures which controlled or eliminated house-dust mite) produced initial relief of symptoms, but became ineffective after six months. The costs of mattress and pillow covers outweighed the benefits.

Allergy workload

An unpublished survey of 30 general practitioners' and 30 practice nurses' perceptions of allergy workload showed that the number of allergy patients seen

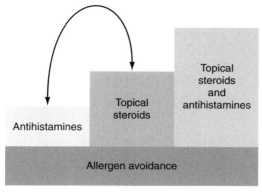

- Immunotherapy for selected patients with immunglobulin E-mediated disease

- Surgery for specific indications for relief of obstruction

+ role of LTRAs

FIGURE 2   Stepwise approach to treatment of perennial rhinitis
Adapted from Mackay, 1998 [11]

TABLE 2   Strength of evidence for treatments of rhinitis. A = directly based on category I evidence (Ia: evidence for meta-analysis of randomized controlled trials; Ib evidence from at least one randomised controlled trial); D = based on category 4 evidence (evidence from expert committee reports or opinions or clinical experience of respected authorities, or both).
Reproduced from ARIA guidelines [15]

Intervention	Seasonal allergic conjunctivitis		Perennial allergic conjunctivitis	
	Adult	Children	Adult	Children
Oral H_1-antihistamine	A	A	A	A
Intranasal H_1-antihistamine	A	A	A	A
Intranasal corticosteroid	A	A	A	A
Intranasal cromone	A	A	A	A
Subcutaneous specific immunotherapy	A	A	A	A
Sublingual or nasal specific immunotherapy	A	A	A	
Allergen avoidance	D	D	D	D

throughout the UK varied widely and was typically dependent on the type of allergy considered. On average, general practitioners see 5–10 allergy cases a week, with an increase in numbers in the spring and summer. The biggest group of patients comprises those with allergic rhinitis (perennial and seasonal), with numbers of patients with hay fever peaking in the spring and summer months. Eczema, urticaria and seasonal allergic asthma are also seen regularly, especially by asthma nurses.

Contact dermatitis and more specific allergies are seen less frequently — a general practitioner might see four or five cases of contact dermatitis per year.

Summary

The population perceives allergy as a common disease, with allergic conjunctivitis viewed as part of seasonal allergic rhinitis or intermittent rhinitis. Reasonably effective remedies are available on prescription and over the counter. Allergy is generally managed in primary care, but general practitioners would benefit from more education and service provision.

References

1. Fraser RC, editor. *Clinical methods: a general practice approach.* Oxford: Butterworth-Heinemann, 1993.

2. Table E1: actual expenditure on the NHS, 1998–99. In: Department of Health. *Health and personal social services statistics. England.* London: Department of Health, 1999. (www.doh.gov.uk/HPSSS/TBL_E1.HTM).

3. Unrestricted principals & equivalents GMS and PMS: analysis of patients list size by principals. In: Department of Health. *General and Personal Medical Services Statistics. England and Wales.* London: Department of Health, 2001. (www.doh.gov.uk/public/nhsworkforce/table92001.xls).

4. Cawenberge P. Consensus statement on the treatment of allergic rhinitis. *Allergy* 2000; **55**: 116–32.

5. (NHS) GP consultations: consultations with doctors in the 14 days before interview, by sex and age of person consulting, and by site of consultation London: Department of Health. 2001 (www.doh.gov.uk/public/nhsworkforce/table92001.xls).

6. (NHS) GP consultations: consultations with doctors in the 14 days before interview, by sex and age of person consulting, and by site of consultation. London: Office for National Statistics, 2002 (www.statistics.gov.uk/statbase/Expodata/Spreadsheets/D5433.xls).

7. Worldwide variation in prevalence of symptoms of asthma, allergic rhinoconjunctivitis, and atopic eczema: ISAAC. The International Study of Asthma and Allergies in Childhood (ISAAC) Steering Committee. *Lancet* 1998; **351(9111)**: 1225–32.

8. Austin JB, Kaur B, Anderson HR *et al.* Hay fever, eczema, and wheeze: a nationwide UK study (ISAAC, international study of asthma and allergies in childhood). *Arch Dis Child* 1999; **81(3)**: 225–30.

9. Grant-Casey J, Scadding G, Pereira S *et al.* Good practice in the management of allergic rhinitis in primary care. Poster presented at the 2001 scientific meeting of the British Society of Allergy and Clinical Immunology.

10. Gøtzsche PC, Hammarquist C, Burr M. House dust mite control measures in the management of asthma: meta-analysis. *BMJ* 1998; **317**: 1105–10.

11. British Society of Allergy and Clinical Immunology. *Rhinitis guidelines.* Southampton: British Society of Allergy and Clinical Immunology, 2000.

12. Mackay IS, Durham SR. ABC of allergies: perennial rhinitis. *BMJ* 1998; **316**: 917–20.

13. Meltzer RO, Malmstom K, Lu S *et al.* Concomitant montelukast and loratadine as a treatment for seasonal allergic rhinitis: a placebo controlled trial. *J Allergy Clin Immunol* 2000; **105(5)**: 917–22.

14. British Society of Allergy and Clinical Immunology. *National Health Service allergy clinics. 2001–2002.* Southampton: British Society of Allergy and Clinical Immunology, 2001.

15. Shekelle PG, Woolf SH, Eccles M, Grimshaw J. Clinical guidelines: developing guidelines. *BMJ* 1999; **318**: 593–6.

Panel discussion

MARTIN CHURCH: You mentioned that desensitization is no longer used because of a problem with it around 10–15 years ago when there were some deaths. That initiated the legal requirement for a two-hour wait after desensitization before the patient could be released, but the requirement had been decreased to one hour. What is the situation now?

DERMOT RYAN: Desensitization is allowed if the general practitioner has full resuscitation equipment and has taken an advanced resuscitation course, which means that it is not done in primary care.

MARTIN CHURCH: Desensitization is used a lot in the USA and continental Europe, but here it is used for cat allergies only in hospital and not often for house-dust mites. Do you recommend it for anything?

DERMOT RYAN: Occasionally I send patients to see the allergist, but the waiting time is at least 18 months (if you have a service in your area). This means that we tend to refer those with anaphylactic or anaphylactoid reactions rather than those who require desensitization.

MARTIN CHURCH: Desensitization probably works by eliciting immune tolerance — possibly by increasing immunoglobulin G_4 levels to develop immune tolerance rather than by inhibiting any substances.

DERMOT RYAN: Researchers on the continent are working on sublingual desensitization.

DAVID EASTY: The problem with serious cases is that the patients are sensitive to so many allergens that desensitization to one allergen makes no difference.

MARK ABELSON: No evidence shows that desensitization works or that it makes allergy worse. We have 'desensitized' patients in a controlled setting by putting pollen in various concentrations in the same patient's eyes over many years. I have been treating some patients for up to 20 years and we have put pollen in their eye hundreds of times, yet they continue to respond. We have also looked at a group of patients who were initially desensitized in season and we did not see any differences — to the point that we do not restrict desensitization in clinical trials. Additionally we did two studies on anti-immunoglobulin E (IgE) — one systemically and one topically, over the years no effect was seen.

DERMOT RYAN: If you were looking at seasonal allergic conjunctivitis in isolation, the cost involved in desensitizing a patient systemically would far outweigh the benefits and would not be economically viable in this country.

JAMES McGILL: It is such a mild disease that it can be controlled with drops, such as mast cell stabilizers (eg nedocromil or lodoxamide) or H_1 blockers (eg levocabastine or azelastine), so it is not worth pursuing desensitization.

MARTIN CHURCH: The possible use of anti-IgE is again restricted by the cost-effectiveness in general practice for this disease.

DERMOT RYAN: Loratadine is no longer available as a prescription medication for people 12 years of age and older, although it is still available for purchase over the counter at a pharmacy [1].

MARK ABELSON: The concordance between skin and ocular challenges in the same individuals is interesting: up to 25% of 3000–4000 patients we have tested did not repond to ocular challenge although they were skin-test positive.

MARTIN CHURCH: I agree that the expression of an allergic disease in a given organ is individual-dependent, but the use of a skin test is not an indicator of allergic disease, it just confirms the presence of circulating IgE. For example, I have high levels of IgE, typically to house-dust mite, but I have never had an allergic disease. Many patients with very low levels of allergen have a 'weakness' in an organ, so they may have asthma, rhinitis, seasonal allergic conjunctivitis or atopic dermatitis. Skin tests do not necessarily predict allergies.

MARK ABELSON: Perhaps we are saying that awareness of the clinical manifestations, such as itching, redness and swelling, and when they occur, is critical to the diagnosis in a particular individual and to assigning appropriate diagnosis and therapy. The most important thing in determining whether the symptoms are caused by allergy is to ask patients if their eyes itch.

DERMOT RYAN: I think it is important to treat the individual based on the symptoms present and not on the tests. Skin prick tests may be falsely positive or falsely negative — at best, a positive test indicates only a propensity not a certainty for atopic disease.

MARTIN CHURCH: We should clarify that atopy is the ability to produce IgE and show a positive skin test, while allergy is an expression of a disease using the IgE produced. For an allergy to be expressed, we suspect that there has also to be a 'weakness' in the target organ. For example, a genetic polymorphism has been found in over 50% of asthmatics which is thought to be associated with hypertrophy of bronchial smooth muscle [2]. Once IgE is produced by the allergic response, people with such a lung 'weakness' are at risk of developing asthma. At the University of Southampton, UK, we are working on a theory that something abnormal about the epidermal cells of the conjunctiva allows allergen penetration in people with allergic conjunctivitis but not in people without the disease.

DAVID EASTY: Dr Ryan, do you have complications when you use steroids for nasal symptoms and do you see perennial nasal rhinitis?

DERMOT RYAN: There are two possible types of complication with nasal steroids: systemic and local. Most local steroids will produce adverse effects if used for long enough, with some atrophy of the mucous membrane and localized bleeding. With newer nasal steroids — fluticasone and mometasone — systemic absorption is negligible and they can be used liberally. The older steroids have much greater systemic bioavailability and in patients with rhinitis who are also taking steroids through another route, it is possible to produce systemic overload. We see a certain number of patients with perennial nasal rhinitis, although it is not as common as seasonal allergic rhinitis. Such patients take treatment for a period of time, feel well, stop it and return after six weeks because the symptoms have returned — perhaps they limit their own systemic absorption of steroids by their 'on–off' use.

JAMES McGILL: You talk about allergen checking, and I think history is vital. In the USA, ragwort is the important allergen; in the UK, pollen is important in rural areas, but in towns, the house-dust mite is more important because air conditioning means that windows tend to stay closed.

MARK ABELSON: Professor Blackley in 1873 was aware of geographic discrepancies with respect to those living in rural and urban areas [3]. There is a growing consensus for the adjuvant effects of hydrocarbon emissions and particularly the pollutants that may exacerbate allergic responses in certain environments [4].

MARTIN CHURCH: It is interesting that you mention Charles Blackley — he first commented on the hygiene theory of allergy, a theory which was revived by Erica von Mutius, who studied children from farms and cities and found exactly the same difference over 100 years later [5]. The major problems with respect to pollution are the diesel particles, the so-called PM10s, which stick to pollen grains and other allergens. Some evidence suggests that this increases the irritancy of the local surface of the allergen and enables it to dissolve through the stigma and style to deliver the gamete to the ovary of the plant [6].

MARK ABELSON: The portal of entry component of the allergen — how it gets into the systemic system — could be enhanced by irritants.

MARTIN CHURCH: Pollution facilitates and exacerbates entry of the pollen, but it does not cause the problem.

DAVID EASTY: The literature used to state that patients with parasitic or helminthic disease in Africa failed to develop atopy or allergy.

MARTIN CHURCH: The theory is that patients produce large amounts of IgE during parasite infestation, so the small amount of IgE produced in response to house-dust mites is insignificant.

MARK ABELSON: Professor Pat Nuttall from the Institute of Biology at Oxford, UK, identified that tick saliva contained components of histamine-binding protein and stabilizing agents that prevent us from being aware of the tick's presence on the body by suppressing any allergic response. This substance is being evaluated as a potential anti-allergic remedy.

DERMOT RYAN: Seasonal allergic conjunctivitis taken in isolation is extremely rare — it almost always occurs in conjunction with seasonal allergic rhinitis. The other eye disorders that have been discussed are so rare that most general practitioners would not encounter them. The history would be entirely different: somebody with seasonal allergic conjunctivitis or rhinitis generally presents within a week or two of the onset of symptoms and they have classic symptoms that last for more than a few days. The first course of action would be a trial of treatment: if eye symptoms and itching are predominant, treatment would initially be with an antihistamine and if nasal symptoms are predominant, initial treatment would be with a nasal steroid. If neither approach controls the symptoms individually, then the treatments would be combined. Our survey included over 300 general practitioners and 85% applied this management approach because they want simple solutions [7].

DAVID EASTY: Did you ask whether general practitioners actually examine the eye in these cases?

DERMOT RYAN: We did not, but I can almost guarantee that no general practitioner does because there is not enough time for the detailed examination you described. When it is appropriate, general practitioners examine the eyes. For example, many practices perform an ophthalmology examination as part of the management of patients with diabetes, but others will send them to an optician, an eye clinic or an eye-screening service. Most general practitioners' skills in using an ophthalmoscope are really quite limited — myself included — whereas opticians have had three years' training. If I have a concern I refer the patient to an optician initially, because it will be four or five months before they see an ophthalmologist. The principle is similar to cardiology, for example — I do not need to know how to do an echocardiogram, rather I need to know where to send a patient to have it done.

References

1. Adelroth E, Rak S, Haahtela T et al. Recombinant humanized mAb-E25, an anti-IgE mAb, in birch pollen-induced seasonal allergic rhinitis. J Allergy Clin Immunol 2000; **106**: 253–9.

2. Van Eerdewegh P, Little RD, Dupuis J et al. Association of the ADAM33 gene with asthma and bronchial hyperresponsiveness. Nature 2002; **418**: 426–30.

3. Blackley CH. On hay-fever. Oxford: Oxford Historical Books, 1873.

4. Anderson HR, Ponce de Leon A, Bland JM et al. Air pollution, pollens, and daily admissions for asthma in London 1987–92. Thorax 1998; **53(10)**: 842–8.

5. Von Mutius E. Environmental factors influencing the development and progression of pediatric asthma. J Allergy Clin Immunol 2002; **109**: S525–32.

6. D'Amato G, Liccardi G, D'Amato M, Cazzola M. Outdoor air pollution, climatic changes and allergic bronchial asthma. Eur Respir J 2002; **20**: 763–76.

7. Grant-Casey J, Scadding G, Pereira S et al. Good practice in the management of allergic rhinitis in primary care. Poster presented at the 2001 scientific meeting of the British Society of Allergy and Clinical Immunology.

Mechanisms of allergy and implications for treatment

Martin Church

Seasonal allergic conjunctivitis is primarily a mast cell-mediated allergic response. The offending allergens are plant pollens or fungal spores and the clinical symptoms occur only during the seasons in which high atmospheric concentrations of these allergens are reached.

Mechanisms of allergic response

In susceptible individuals, exposure to pollen grains or fungal spores stimulates the immune system to produce immunoglobuin E (IgE) antibodies. Immunoglobulin E is unique in that it binds to a variety of inflammatory cells. Of particular relevance to seasonal allergic conjunctivitis is the ability of IgE to 'prime' mast cells in the conjunctiva by binding to high-affinity receptors on the cell surface. Further exposure to allergen activates 'primed' mast cells to release preformed and newly generated mediators [1]. Of these, histamine is the most pertinent to seasonal allergic conjunctivitis, as by stimulating histamine H_1-receptors, it is responsible for

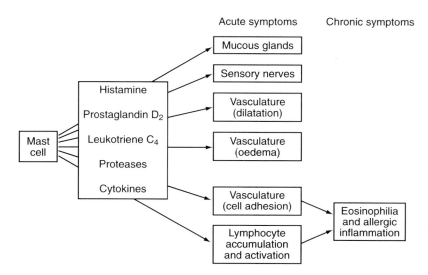

FIGURE I   Cell responses and symptoms in seasonal allergic conjunctivitis

producing most of the troublesome symptoms (Figure 1). These include lacrimation (tear formation), sensory nerve stimulation (itch), vasodilatation (reddening of the conjunctiva) and chemosis (local oedema) (Figure 2) [2]. Mast cells produce many other mediators in addition to histamine (Figure 1). Leukotriene C_4 (LTC_4) plays a major role in asthma through its potent ability to contract bronchial smooth muscle, but appears to have little effect on the cells present in the conjunctiva. The mast cell proteases, tryptase and chymase, and the mast-cell cytokines, including interleukin-4 (IL-4), IL-5 and granulocyte-macrophage colony-stimulating factor (GM-CSF) are responsible for initiating and maintaining allergic inflammation and, as such, are of more importance in chronic allergic conditions, eg vernal conjunctivitis.

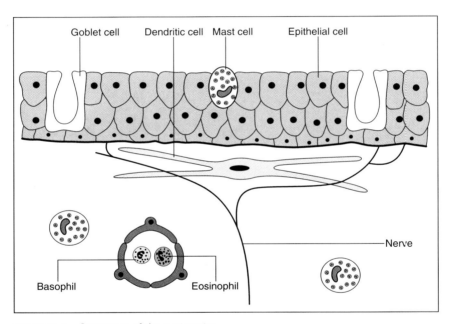

FIGURE 2 Structures of the conjunctiva

Drugs for the treatment of seasonal allergic conjunctivitis and rhinoconjunctivitis

From the above, we may construct a working model of the pathogenetic mechanism of seasonal allergic conjunctivitis—interaction of mast cell-derived histamine with histamine H_1-receptors on glands, sensory nerves and blood vessels is responsible for the symptoms of seasonal allergic conjunctivitis. Interestingly, the same working model may be used for seasonal allergic rhinitis. In seasonal allergic rhinitis, the interaction of histamine with histamine H_1-receptors on glands results in rhinorrhoea, on sensory nerves causes sneezing and on blood vessels is partly responsible for nasal blockage. As seasonal allergic rhinitis and seasonal allergic conjunctivitis have similar pathogenetic mechanisms and commonly present together as rhinoconjunctivitis [2, 3], it is pertinent to consider their drug therapy together.

Drugs may influence the mechanistic cascade of seasonal allergic conjunctivitis and seasonal allergic rhinitis in several different ways:

- prevention of activation of histamine H_1-receptors using H_1-antihistamines
- inhibition of mast-cell activation by the so-called mast cell-stabilizing drugs, nedocromil sodium and lodoxamide
- inhibition of the migration and maturation of mast cells by corticosteroids, thereby reducing the number of mast cells in the conjunctival and nasal mucosae.

Antihistamines

Four quite distinct receptors exist for histamine [4]. As mentioned above, stimulation of histamine H_1-receptors on mucous glands, sensory nerves and blood vessels is responsible for most of the symptoms of seasonal allergic conjunctivitis and seasonal allergic rhinitis. In addition, their presence on smooth muscle contributes to the symptoms of intestinal allergy. Histamine H_2-receptors are associated mainly with gastric secretion although they are also associated with some immunomodulatory actions. Histamine H_3-receptors are mainly associated with nerves, particularly in the central nervous system, where they appear to be neuroprotective. Recently, studies of the genome have revealed a fourth histamine receptor, the H_4-receptor. Although we know little of the function of this receptor, it seems to be present on eosinophils and on some precursors of inflammatory cells in the bone marrow. For symptomatic relief in seasonal allergic conjunctivitis and seasonal allergic rhinitis, H_1-antihistamines are the antihistamines of choice, as H_2- and H_3-antihistamines afford little protection.

Systemic antihistamines are generally used for the treatment of seasonal allergic rhinitis, with or without seasonal allergic conjunctivitis. Topical antihistamines, on the other hand, are generally used to treat seasonal allergic conjunctivitis alone. or as an adjunct to systemic therapy when the ocular symptoms are particularly troublesome. However, there is a school of thought that the redistribution of topical antihistamine throughout the nasopharynx after ocular administration may also help to relieve the symptoms of rhinitis.

Systemic H$_1$-antihistamines

First-generation H$_1$-antihistamines, such as chlorpheniramine, are still available for the systemic treatment of rhinoconjunctivitis. Their great advantage is their cheapness and their great disadvantages are their anticholinergic effects and ability to cause drowsiness. If administered at night, however, these disadvantages may actually be advantageous.

Second-generation H$_1$-antihistamines are largely free of anticholinergic and sedative properties. Because of their capacity to relieve nasal and ocular symptoms, their favourable risk:benefit ratio at standard clinical doses and their satisfactory pharmacokinetics, the second-generation antihistamines can be considered as the first-choice treatment for allergic rhinoconjunctivitis as far as disease severity and symptoms are concerned [5]. A wide variety of second-generation antihistamines is on the market today, but it is not the role of this paper to recommend any one above the others. A few general comments regarding these drugs and their usage include:

- Although all H$_1$-antihistamines have a similar basic pharmacological profile, they are remarkably different from each other in many respects — both pharmacodynamically and pharmacokinetically. Pharmacodynamic differences include the characteristics and duration of the binding of the drugs to their receptors. Pharmacokinetic differences include bioavailability, volume of distribution, degree of protein binding and plasma half-life. Even the route of clearance may differ, eg desloratadine is metabolized extensively to inactive products in the liver, whereas almost all levocetirizine is excreted unchanged through the kidney. These differences underlie what many practicing clinicians know well: some antihistamines suit some patients appropriately while other drugs suit other patients.

- If we were prescribing, for example, an antibiotic for someone with severe pneumonia, we might consider giving a loading dose in order to reach steady state conditions rapidly; because the most effective treatment should be delivered as quickly as possible. Why not consider doing the same with anti-histamines when your patient stands in front of you with nose streaming and eyes itching intolerably? Again, the most effective treatment as quickly as possible is what is needed. Table I shows that with an antihistamine whose half-life is approximately 24 hours, it takes over five days to reach steady state levels (when the drug levels are approximately twice those achieved after the first dose). However, if a double dose is given to start with, steady state is achieved immediately. In practice, it may be better to give one tablet immediately and the second at bedtime just in case of any sedative effects at the onset of treatment.

- H_1-antihistamines have been claimed to have anti-inflammatory actions. This will be discussed in more detail when describing the effects of topical antihistamines in the eye (see Page 30). However, it is pertinent to note here that any such properties are unlikely to contribute to their efficacy in relieving the symptoms of rhinoconjunctivitis.
- It has also been claimed that the active metabolites of previous second-generation antihistamines, such as fexofenadine, are third-generation antihistamines. However, a recent study group of the European Academy of Allergy and Clinical Immunology recommended that the use of such a term implied a clinical advantage over second-generation drugs. As such, the term 'third-generation antihistamine' should be reserved for drugs with a significant clinical advantage over current drugs. At present, no drugs meet this criterion and, as such, all the H_1-antihistamines on the market today are 'second-generation antihistamines' (unpublished data).

TABLE I   The effect of a loading dose on systemic levels of any given drug

| Day | Without loading dose | | With loading dose | |
	Daily accumulation	Peak level	Daily accumulation	Peak level
1	32	32	2×32	64
2	32 + 16	48	32 + 32	64
3	32 + 16 + 8	56	32 + 16 + 16	64
4	32 + 16 + 8 + 4	60	32 + 16 + 8 + 8	64
5	32 + 16 + 8 + 4 + 2	62	32 + 16 + 8 + 4 + 4	64

This table gives an example of how a loading dose may influence the time taken by a drug to reach steady kinetics. The assumptions made are (a) that the drug has a half-life of 24 hours; (b) that it is given as a once daily medication; (c) one tablet gives a peak plasma level of 32 ng/ml, and (d) two tablets are given as a loading dose.

Topical H_1-antihistamines

In addition to systemic administration, antihistamines such as azelastine, emedastine or levocabastine, may be given topically, either for the treatment of seasonal allergic conjunctivitis in isolation or in addition to systemic therapy when necessary.

To understand a little more about its mechanism(s) of action, we examined the effects of levocabastine in an allergen challenge model of seasonal allergic conjunctivitis [6]. Treatment twice daily for two weeks was very effective in relieving the symptoms of itch, hyperaemia and tearing following challenge. Assay of mast cell-derived mediators in the tears showed no reduction in histamine or prostaglandin D_2 (PGD_2) release compared with placebo. However, expression of the adhesion protein intercellular adhesion molecule-1 (ICAM-1) on the vascular endothelium was reduced.

These results bring into question the so-called anti-inflammatory actions of H_1-antihistamines. In order to put such effects on a scientific basis, a recent review by Leurs *et al* postulated that some anti-inflammatory effects of H_1-antihistamines are subsequent to their interaction with H_1-receptors, while others are receptor-independent [7]. The receptor-independent actions, including inhibition of mast cell- and basophil-mediator release, necessitate high concentrations of drug and are unlikely to contribute to the beneficial therapeutic effects of antihistamines in the treatment of allergic diseases. This was confirmed by the above studies [6]. However, the receptor-dependent anti-inflammatory effects, including downregulation of ICAM-1 expression, are demonstrable at therapeutic concentrations of drug and appear to correspond with the potency at the H_1-receptor [7]. But what is their clinical relevance? Probably very little in the treatment of seasonal allergic conjunctivitis and other 'acute' allergic responses in which there is little accumulation of inflammatory cells.

Mast cell-stabilizing drugs

Seasonal allergic conjunctivitis may also be treated by topical administration of the so-called 'mast cell-stabilizing drugs', such as nedocromil sodium, lodoxamide and sodium cromoglycate [8].

To understand more about mechanism(s) of action of drugs of this type, we again used the allergen challenge model of seasonal allergic conjunctivitis [6]. As with levocabastine, treatment with nedocromil sodium twice daily for two weeks was very effective in relieving symptoms of itch, hyperaemia and tearing after challenge. Examination of the tears showed significant reductions of histamine or PGD_2, suggesting 'mast cell stabilization' to be levocabastine's mechanism of action. However, this study also revealed a novel finding. Six hours after challenge, the late phase response brought about a second rise in the severity of symptoms and a second rise in tear levels of histamine. Again, nedocromil sodium relieved the symptoms; however, it did not reduce histamine levels in the tears, which at this time are probably basophil derived. So how did nedocromil sodium provide symptomatic relief? Subsequent research showed it to be prevention of sensory nerve activation by an effect on chloride channels [9].

Nedocromil sodium and related drugs are also suggested to have anti-inflammatory effects, even though we found no effect on adhesion protein expression [6]. However, in seasonal allergic conjunctivitis — a relatively mild allergic condition — an anti-inflammatory action of a drug is not a prerequisite, as there is little influx and activation of secondary inflammatory cells such as neutrophils and eosinophils. In the more severe vernal conjunctivitis, where the influx of such cells leads to secondary conjunctival damage, nedocromil sodium has been shown to reduce significantly the number of neutrophils and eosinophils in the tears [10].

Corticosteroids

Corticosteroids are the most effective anti-inflammatory drugs available and yet one of the most feared because of their unwanted effects. To use them properly, it is necessary to understand a little of their mechanism(s) of action and pharmacokinetics.

All glucocorticoids have the same mechanism of action at the cellular level. Essentially they have intracellular actions. After their association with the plasma membrane of cells, glucocorticoids combine with intracellular receptors, which they activate. The activated receptor then translocates to the nucleus, where it modulates the effects of the transcription factors nuclear factor-κB (NF-κB) and activator protein-1 (AP-1), which are involved in the production of many pro-inflammatory adhesion proteins, cytokines, chemokines and growth factors. Alternatively, it stimulates the production of ribonucleases, which destabilize the messenger RNA for selected cytokines. Although it is not the place of this short review to go into great detail about the pharmacodynamics and pharmacokinetics of corticosteroids, the following points may help in the appreciation of their strengths and weaknesses in the treatment of allergic diseases:

- As corticosteroids have an essentially intracellular action, their actions are not readily demonstrable for 12–24 hours. At this time, cytokine production will be reduced as will the development of inflammation. However, it will take considerably longer, perhaps even months, for established inflammation to regress.
- Corticosteroids do not inhibit mast cell degranulation and cannot, as such, prevent the onset of an early-phase allergic response. However, by inhibiting the production of stem cell factor, a product of the transcription factor NF-κB, corticosteroids reduce the number of mast cells within tissues. This effect is slow to become apparent because of the slow turnover of mast cells. For example, it took three weeks of topical treatment with clobetasol to reduce the number of dermal mast cells by 50% [11]. As a consequence, the most appropriate use of corticosteroids is as a topical intranasal prophylactic treatment for seasonal rhinoconjunctivitis. For this use, treatment should be initiated around one month before the expected onset of hay fever. Similar topical use in the eye is not recommended due to the unwanted effects described on Page 32.

- Although not pertinent to seasonal allergic conjunctivitis, the anti-inflammatory actions of corticosteroids in inhibiting eosinophils' accumulation and activation in vernal conjunctivitis may be sight-saving.
- The unwanted effects of topical corticosteroid administration to the nose are negligible, as evidenced by the availability of such preparations 'over the counter'. The local immunosuppressive effects of topical administration of corticosteroids to the eye will aggravate dendritic ulceration caused by the herpes simplex virus. Topical administration of corticosteroids to the eye may also precipitate 'steroid-induced' glaucoma in predisposed individuals. Both of these conditions may be sight-threatening. The mobilization of proteins that may precipitate in the cornea means that both topical steroids and high doses of systemic corticosteroids may cause cataract formation (steroid cataract).
- The pharmacokinetics of corticosteroids intended for systemic and topical use differs markedly. Drugs intended for systemic use, such as prednisolone, are readily absorbed from the gastrointestinal tract, distributed widely throughout the body and have a relatively long duration of action. Corticosteroids intended for topical use, such as beclometasone and fluticasone, are poorly absorbed through mucosal membranes and from the gastrointestinal tract. Fluticasone has an added advantage in that any drug which is absorbed systemically is metabolized rapidly by the liver.

Summary

Both seasonal allergic conjunctivitis and seasonal allergic rhinitis are primarily mast cell-dependent, immediate-type allergic responses. Symptomatic relief may be afforded by H_1-antihistamines given orally for seasonal allergic rhinitis and topically for seasonal allergic conjunctivitis. Mast cell stabilizers, such as nedocromil sodium and lodoxamide, are also effective topical treatments for seasonal allergic conjunctivitis. Topical corticosteroids are safe and effective prophylactic drugs for seasonal allergic rhinitis, but they should be used with caution in the eye.

References

1. O'Byrne PM, Persson CGA, Church MK. Cellular and mediator mechanisms of the early phase allergic response. In: Holgate ST, Church MK, Lichtenstein LM, eds. *Allergy*. London: Mosby, 2001: 325–36.

2. Lightman S, Buckley RJ, Hingorani M. Conjunctivitis. In: Holgate ST, Church MK, Lichtenstein LM, eds. *Allergy*. London: Mosby, 2001: 77–92.

3. Scadding GK, Church MK. Rhinitis. In: Holgate ST, Church MK, Lichtenstein LM, eds. *Allergy*. London: Mosby, 2001: 55–76.

4. Church MK. H_1-antihistamines and inflammation. *Clin Exp Allergy* 2001; **31**: 1341–3.

5. van Cauwenberge P, Bachert C, Passalacqua G *et al*. Consensus statement on the treatment of allergic rhinitis. *European Academy of Allergology and Clinical Immunology Allergy* 2000; **55**: 116–34.

6. Ahluwalia P, Anderson DF, Wilson SJ et al. Nedocromil sodium and levocabastine reduce the symptoms of conjunctival allergen challenge by different mechanisms. J Allergy Clin Immunol 2001; **108**: 449–54.

7. Leurs R, Church MK, Taglialatela M. H_1-antihistamines: inverse agonism, anti-inflammatory actions and cardiac effects. Clin Exp Allergy 2002; **32**: 489–98.

8. Church MK, Makino S. Drugs for the treatment of allergic disease. In: Holgate ST, Church MK, Lichtenstein LM, eds. Allergy. London: Mosby, 2001: 353–70.

9. Ahluwalia P, McGill JI, Church MK. Nedocromil sodium inhibits histamine-induced itch and flare in human skin. Br J Pharmacol 2001; **132**: 613–5.

10. Bonini S, Barney NP, Schiavone M et al. Effectiveness of nedocromil sodium 2% eyedrops on clinical symptoms and tear fluid cytology of patients with vernal conjunctivitis. Eye 1992; **6**: 648–52.

11. Cole ZA, Clough GF, Church MK. Inhibition by glucocorticoids of the mast cell-dependent weal and flare response in human skin in vivo. Br J Pharmacol 2001; **132**: 286–92.

Discussion

MARK ABELSON: The shield ulcers seen in vernal conjunctivitis contain Charcot-Leyden crystals that are seen on electron microscopy and in assays for eosinophil major basic protein. This means that the system of remodelling you described impacts on the ocular surface and produces serious clinical manifestations. This response causes damage and can eventually result in scarring, the size of which depends on the stage of the disease. I think it would be realistic to look at some of the keratitis we occasionally see in patients with more severe seasonal atopy as a minor manifestation of the same component of eosinophil activation.

JAMES McGILL: I agree because the pH of tears is completely altered in patients with severe allergic disease. I think that is caused by the eosinophilic content of the tears—so the tears become hyperosmotic, which leads to changes in the corneal epithelium, causing erosions and therefore keratitis.

MARK ABELSON: Your results with nedocromil sodium in skin are fascinating. When prostaglandins and leukotriene C_4, D_4 and E_4 were first uncovered in the 1980s and were available as compounds, I put some leukotriene C_4 in my eye. It produced no clinical manifestations. The highest concentration of D_4 also had no reaction in my eye.

MARTIN CHURCH: We have the same experiences in the skin. Prostaglandin D_2 and leukotriene C_4 have very small effects at concentrations far in excess of those they would ever reach naturally in the target tissue.

MARK ABELSON: I think they probably play a role downstream, in combination with many other things or other diseases, but I think certainly in seasonal allergy in the eye, their role may be limited in the acute setting.

MARTIN CHURCH: I'm often asked whether we should be using desloratadine and levocetirizine rather than the generic loratadine and cetirizine, which are now off patent.

DERMOT RYAN: It is important to note that desloratadine is the only available prescription for people aged >12 years and that loratadine has been discontinued as a prescription drug and is available only over the counter in the United Kingdom. I saw your slide, Professor Church, on loading doses for antihistamines during your talk and was very impressed by it; I will change my clinical practice as a resut of it, ie by advising my patients to take two tablets on day one and one a day thereafter.

JAMES McGILL: Professor Church, you said that it took days for corticosteroids to get working on the mast cells.

MARTIN CHURCH: The life of a mast cell is about six weeks, so you will reduce their numbers by about 50% in 3–4 weeks.

JAMES McGILL: Yet when we have severe vernal conjunctivitis, we use up to hourly steroids, which seem to work quickly. Do you think there is a washout effect? Have there been any placebo-controlled trials for vernal conjunctivitis for steroids *versus* placebo?

MARK ABELSON: There is no good study, but the clinical evidence clearly shows that within 24 hours of reasonably high doses — usually prednisolone acetate 1% six or eight times a day — there is a dramatic response. I agree with Professor Church that, at this stage, we're largely looking at stabilization of eosinophils. The eosinophils are bound to ICAM receptors and the epithelial surface, and release keratitis-producing substances; I think this is the effect we are seeing. When we taper the dose, we are trying to keep the eosinophils under control and to decrease the likelihood of a pool of mast cells being increased.

JAMES McGILL: Should we be starting our patients with vernal conjunctivitis on steroids in March rather than April?

MARK ABELSON: I think it is best to.

JAMES McGILL: Do you start them off with steroids before the season comes in? I maintain them on a mast cell stabilizer over the winter and they sometimes have no symptoms.

DAVID EASTY: I ensure that such patients have a bottle of steroids in their refrigerator, so that as soon as they become symptomatic, they use the steroids — that's almost prophylactic.

JAMES McGILL: But that will take time to kick in: they ought to be starting before they get symptoms. It would be nice to compare the control in patients treated prophylactically and those treated symptomatically.

DAVID EASTY: Professor Church, have you performed dose–response studies in your challenge models to determine whether steroids at different concentrations have different effects on the inflammatory processes and immunological changes that you've identified?

MARTIN CHURCH: Most of my work has been in the skin looking at clobetasol.

DAVID EASTY: Does the skin respond in different ways to different concentrations of steroids?

MARTIN CHURCH: I think the answer probably would be yes — but concentration, bioavailability and effect do not always increase in parallel.

MARK ABELSON: We used a dose–response mechanism to determine the most effective concentrations for lodopredanol and rimexolone [1]. We also looked at strong steroids, such as prednisolone acetate, in different formulations, and we saw a plateau of effect based on some of Professor Church's mechanisms. The amount of effect is very small. To maximize the effect, we used a tobramycin and dexamethasone ophthalmic suspension for two, four and six weeks to find the optimal loading period, which was around four weeks. The other point is that steroids seem to have a separate effect in terms of vasoconstrictive effects, and studies are using laser Doppler to determine the bioequivalence of steroids on the skin related to the amount of vasoconstriction. There seems to be a separate function that manifests itself and is detectable in ocular challenge models.

DAVID EASTY: Did you get effects with much lower concentrations of steroids than are normally used?

MARK ABELSON: We found that fluorometholone was very similar in effect to the more expensive newer steroids, but then we found the optimal doses and the concentration range, which gave a better risk:benefit ratio.

MARTIN CHURCH: Is there a steroid eye drop that contains one of the new non-absorbed steroids, like fluticasone or budesonide? The steroids cited in the British National Formulary will all be absorbed straight through the cornea and cause glaucoma problems.

DAVID EASTY: We use fluorometholone and clobetasone as, according to our literature, they do not raise the intraocular pressure (IOP).

MARTIN CHURCH: They pass quickly through the cornea, and they do ra se the pressure in clinical practice [2]. This is why I wonder whether treatment patterns might change if fluticasone was available as eye drops.

MARK ABELSON: We have no reason to assume that corticosteroids act on a different receptor to produce inflammation than to elevate IOP. We hope there is, but current evidence suggests not.

MARTIN CHURCH: What we're looking at now is whether the drug reaches the receptor: if the drug is not absorbed systemically, as with fluticasone, it may not actually reach the receptor to cause the problem.

DERMOT RYAN: Fluticasone is absorbed systemically [3, 4]. When it is administered orally, 99.5% of it is inactivated by first-pass metabolism through the liver; but it still has systemic activity because when given for asthma, 10% is absorbed through the lung and exerts some systemic effects.

MARK ABELSON: No evidence for any steroid given in any way has shown that the effect of its concentration with regard to inflammation can be decoupled from its IOP-elevating effect if it is delivered to the eye. The effectiveness in inflammation of all of the agents given at different concentrations runs absolutely in parallel with their IOP-elevating effects — it is a good way of determining their intraocular absorption. Nothing unique about the eye pharmacokinetically suggests that the effects can be decoupled.

MARTIN CHURCH: Talking very briefly about leukotriene antagonists, results from certain other conditions, particularly atopic dermatitis, asthma and even rhinitis, show that a proportion of individuals actually benefits from addition of systemic drugs, such as montelukast — the leukotriene C_4/D_4 antagonist [5]. Recent studies showed that people who respond to leukotriene C_4/D_4 antagonists have a genetic polymorphism: a T to C conversion in chromosome 5 [6], so we can now genetically type people who may respond to these drugs. The polymorphism allows a second transcription factor to act on the synthetic process of leukotriene C_4, thereby increasing its efficiency. In some patients, there may be an additional benefit; in many, there will not. Dr Ryan, have you any clinical experience with montelukast?

DERMOT RYAN: I have tried montelukast in 54 or 55 patients altogether — mainly for asthma. In about one-third, I've seen absolutely no response; in another third I've seen some response, particularly with cough; and in one-third, a huge response allows you to reduce other treatments, particularly inhaled steroids. Two patients with seasonal allergic rhinitis who responded to nothing else have had extremely good results with montelukast.

MARTIN CHURCH: It is interesting that you're picking up the same sort of percentages as the polymorphism. About 30–40% possibly — and I wonder whether the conjunctivitis side of rhinoconjunctivitis may benefit too.

DERMOT RYAN: It seemed to. The first patient had tried all combinations of conventional medication: he was taking nasal steroids, antihistamines and anything he could buy over the counter. I suggested he try montelukast for a month. He said it was fantastic: on other drugs, his quality of life on a scale of 0 to 10 was 3 or 4; after montelukast, he rated it as 8. He did not have to stay indoors during the day and he could go out on bright days. The treatment was a transforming event for him and helped both nasal and ocular symptoms.

References

1. Abelson M, Howes J, George M. The conjunctival provocation test model of ocular allergy: utility for assessment of an ocular corticosteroid, loteprednol etabonate. *J Ocul Pharmacol Ther* 1998; **14**: 533.

2. Church MK, Makino S. Drugs for the treatment of allergic disease. In: Holgate ST, Church MK, Lichtenstein LM, eds. *Allergy*. London: Mosby, 2001: 353–70.

3. Grove A, Allam C, McFarlane LC et al. A comparison of the systemic bioactivity of inhaled budesonide and fluticasone propionate in normal subjects. *Br J Clin Pharmacol* 1994; **38(6)**: 527–32.

4. Lipworth BJ, Jackson CM. Safety of inhaled and intranasal corticosteroids. Lessons for the new millennium. *Drug Safety* 2000; **23(1)**: 11–33.

5. Drazen JM, Israel E, O'Byrne PM. Treatment of asthma with drugs modifying the leukotriene pathway. *N Engl J Med* 1999; **340**:197–206.

6. Sampson AP, Siddiqui S, Buchanan D et al. Variant LTC_4 synthase allele modifies cysteinyl leukotriene synthesis in eosinophils and predicts clinical response to zafirlukast. *Thorax* 2000; **55 (Suppl 2)**: S28–31.

Allergic eye disease — steps to treatment

James McGill

The prevalence of allergic diseases — asthma and rhinoconjunctivitis — is increasing in English-speaking countries around the world, such as the UK, Australia and New Zealand, but it is decreasing in other countries, such as Ethiopia, North Africa and India [1–3]. Allergic conditions are more prevalent in Western than Eastern countries and are less common in less developed countries, although their prevalence starts to increase as countries become more developed (Figure 1) [2]. Increases in prevalence in English-speaking countries must be accounted for in part by genetic factors, and this is under investigation [4]. Allergies are more common in urban than rural communities [5].

In the UK, one in ten people are asthmatic and one in three children wheeze. Seasonal allergic conjunctivitis is the most common allergic disease and is present in about 20% of the general population [6]. Perennial allergic conjunctivitis is not as common as seasonal allergic conjunctivitis. The chronic diseases, atopic keratoconjunctivitis and vernal keratoconjunctivitis, are much less prevalent, but they are regularly seen by ophthalmologists because they are a problem to treat and are chronic and sight-threatening [6].

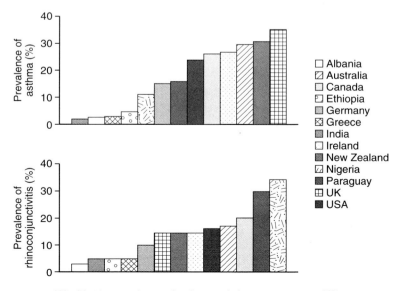

FIGURE 1   Worldwide prevalence of asthma and rhinoconjunctivitis [2]

Cellular mechanisms behind allergic eye disease

The mild allergic diseases — seasonal and perennial allergic conjunctivitis — are driven by mast cells, which are central to the allergic process. These cells store and manufacture the cytokines responsible for the inflammatory cascade. If the mast cells can be controlled, so can the disease. Atopic keratoconjunctivitis, atopic blepharoconjunctivitis, vernal catarrh and giant papillary conjunctivitis are T-cell orchestrated, but mast cell-driven.

Research at the University of Southampton, UK, is investigating how allergens enter the eye: an enzyme contained within the allergen dissolves the epithelial surface to provide an entry point. In the conjunctiva, layers of apical, intermediate and basal cells are held together by hemidesmosomes and by E-cadherin. A tight junction is present at the surface and the cell structure is held together by cytokeratin. Preliminary evidence shows that these proteins are abnormal in atopic patients; the reason for this is unknown, but it may result from repeated disease or it may be an underlying structural abnormality. These changes could allow the allergen to penetrate into the deep tissues and initiate the allergic cascade response. Another way for the allergens to enter is by use of enzymes contained within the allergen that could dissolve the epithelial surface to provide an entry point [7, 8]. Alternatively, the surface contains protease-activated receptors (eg PAR-2), which are underexpressed in atopic patients out of season [9]. Whether these are initiators of the allergic reaction or part of a defence mechanism is not known. Some people have high concentrations of immunoglobulin E in the blood, but they show no evidence of atopic disease. If grass contacts the skin of a non-atopic person, there is no reaction, but if it is injected under the skin, an allergic reaction does occur. This provides evidence of a role for the epithelium in the allergic cascade, especially in its initiation.

The symptoms of seasonal allergic conjunctivitis include red, uncomfortable eyes that itch and water; blurring leads to temporary loss of vision. Many patients have associated allergic diseases. Patients who report sneezing when they dust the house have perennial allergic rhinoconjunctivitis, whereas those whose eyes start itching if they walk outside have seasonal allergic conjunctivitis.

Treatment

The first stage of the treatment of conjunctivitis must involve allergen checking and guidance on avoidance. Therapy includes topical and systemic treatments. Topical treatments include:

- antihistamines (emedastine, levocabastine, azelastine)
- mast cell stabilizers (lodoxamide, nedocromil, sodium cromoglycate)

- vasoconstrictors (antazoline)
- steroids
- ciclosporin.

The antihistamines and vasoconstrictors are fast-acting, the mast cell stabilizers usually take a few days to show an effect and the steroids can take several days to produce any effect [10]. Evidence may support pre-treatment of people with chronic disease that are prone to flare-ups, but for immediate relief, the antihistamines are the treatments of choice [11]. In patients who can predict potential flare-ups, the mast cell stabilizers are extremely effective [12].

Systemic treatments include:

- antihistamines
- steroids
- ciclosporin.

All the systemic agents are slow to act. On the whole, ophthalmologists do not use systemic antihistamines, but patients may be already taking them before referral because of other associated allergic diseases. Although the second-generation antihistamines do not produce sedation, they can produce dry eyes [13]. Therefore topical eye drops, which can be used frequently and effectively, are preferred. Similarly, steroids are used sparingly because of the known side-effects. Ciclosporin has been tested in severe eye disease, but its vehicle is difficult to obtain, it is not stable and it produces side-effects.

Seasonal allergic conjunctivitis

Seasonal allergic conjunctivitis is usually associated with rhinoconjunctivitis and involves an allergic reaction to grass or pollen. It mainly occurs in the spring and summer. Many treatments for seasonal allergic conjunctivitis are available over the counter, including antihistamines, vasoconstrictors and mast cell stabilizers, eg cromoglycate [6, 10]. Hospital eye clinics rarely see patients with seasonal allergic conjunctivitis because the available drugs are usually effective in controlling the patients' symptoms and signs without any known side-effects (except an occasional allergic reaction to the benzalkonium chloride preservatives in the eye drops).

In one study, 0–15 minutes after administration, 50% of patients had symptomatic relief with a mast cell stabilizer, whereas with antihistamines, 100% of patients had a response (Figure 2) [11]. Between 15 and 60 minutes after administration, 60–80% of patients receiving a mast cell stabilizer had a response and still 100% of patients taking antihistamines had a response. This shows that

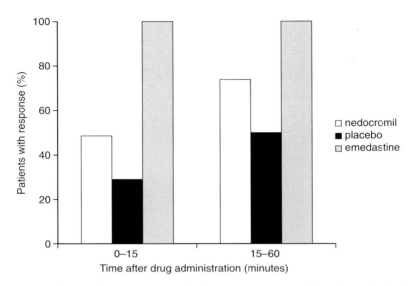

FIGURE 2 Speed of action in seasonal allergic conjunctivitis with nedocromil, placebo and emedastine [11]

antihistamines are the best agents when a fast reaction is needed. Lodoxamide and nedocromil are equally effective when compared with placebo (and more so than cromoglycate) in the treatment of seasonal allergic conjunctivitis [11] and can be used interchangeably.

Perennial allergic conjunctivitis

Perennial allergic conjunctivitis occurs all year round but peaks in the autumn. Patients are allergic to house-dust mites and it is common in office workers and those who live in homes with tightly sealed windows, as air-conditioning aggravates their condition. Many patients have a history of atopy, but they do not necessarily have any systemic disease. This condition is adequately controlled with nedocromil or lodoxamide with respect to both patients' symptom scores and clinical scores [12]. Allergen checking is useful if the history does not reveal an obvious allergen, and guidance on allergen avoidance should be provided. The mast cell stabilizers are excellent, giving a 90% success rate, but their onset of action is slower than that of the antihistamines [13].

Atopic keratoconjunctivitis

Atopic keratoconjunctivitis is commonly seen in hospital clinics after referral by general practitioners. Patients with this condition have severe systemic disease — asthma or atopic dermatitis, especially of the face. They will inevitably have lid involvement. The disease follows a continuous pattern of exacerbations and fluctuations. It is vital to treat the lids because they are full of pathogens. Patients with atopic keratoconjunctivitis develop severe blepharitis and, if meibomium secretions are not produced, the tear film made by the lacrimal gland evaporates, resulting in dry eyes, corneal surface epithelial disorders and ultimately corneal scarring. If scarring spreads to the visual axis, the patient loses their sight. This condition is sight-threatening, chronic and associated with severe diseases, such as herpes simplex, which can be bilateral, devastating and sight-threatering. Keratoconus can also be associated with this condition. Ultimately, many of these patients will need a penetrating corneal graft, whose post-operative care can be can extremely difficult from a management point of view (although not peri-operatively or technically), because of the atopic disease and their reaction to sutures and drugs.

Patients with atopic keratoconjunctivitis should be allergen-checked and advised on allergen avoidance. They are maintained on mast cell stabilizers (nedocromil or lodoxamide) two or three times daily, with steroids used only in acute exacerbations. Such treatment and the recognition of lid disease, which may need systemic tetracycline (one or two tablets of 250 mg oxytetracycline or 100 mg doxycycline a day), will control the condition for many years. The cornea also requires lubrication to prevent epithelial disease as the eyes are often dry. Patients should therefore be prescribed preservative-free drops (too many drops containing preservative have toxic effects on the cornea). People from the Asian and Afro-Asian communities suffer particularly badly with atopic keratoconjunctivitis, and they often need systemic steroids and sometimes ciclosporin.

Patients given systemic steroids are at risk of ocular side-effects such as developing cataracts, glaucoma and sometimes corneal diseases, such as herpes simplex infection or stromal melts.

Herpes simplex corneal infection can be severe, bilateral and sight-threatening. Treatment should be with topical antivirals such as aciclovir, famciclovir or valaciclovir. Once patients have received steroids, they always need to be maintained on topical steroids during a recurrence of herpes simplex. Each time a patient with atopic keratoconjunctivitis presents with a recurrence of herpes simplex, they can be started on antivirals, but they inevitably also will need steroids. Unfortunately, steroids cannot be stopped as soon as the herpes simplex clears up, but must be continued in low doses for 6 months–1 year. Treatment starts with full-strength steroids (prednisolone 0.5% drops) four times a day for a week; the dose is then tapered down monthly; for example, the dose is reduced by half a log dilution to 0.1% four times a day, then by log dilution to 0.03%, then to 0.01%, with an antiviral agent given until 0.01% dilutions of steroid are achieved.

Keratoconus is a problem for patients with atopic keratoconjunctivitis and is difficult to treat. Patients with atopic keratoconjunctivitis have poor long-term visual prognosis: their vision starts to fail and many have corneal surface disease. Lid distortion makes the eyes dry and causes the lids or lashes to rub the cornea, and patients often require lid surgery. Patients often develop glaucoma or cataracts, especially if they have been on topical steroids, and are very difficult to treat — particularly glaucoma, because the conjunctival drainage bleb from the glaucoma surgery becomes blocked up through fibrosis. Cataract surgery is frequently required, but problems with wound healing and infection occur because of lid disease and topical and systemic steroids.

Vernal catarrh or vernal keratoconjunctivitis

Another common condition, although less so in the Caucasian population, is vernal catarrh; it also is known as spring catarrh, because it is worse in the spring. Boys are affected more often than girls until puberty [6, 13]; after puberty, the sex ratio equalizes out — probably because of differences in the sex hormone receptors in the conjunctiva. Vernal keratoconjunctivitis is an interesting disease because it is becoming less common in Caucasians but seems to be increasing in the Asian population. It has two forms:

- the tarsal form, often seen in Caucasians
- the limbal form, with inflammation and swelling around the cornea.

The limbal form is more commonly found in patients of a Mediterranean origin and is more difficult to treat than the tarsal form. In the corneal margin small white spots (Tranta's spots) can occur that are full of eosinophils.

Patients with vernal catarrh should always be allergen-checked because the disease can be sight-threatening if ulcers develop on the central cornea. Such ulcers comprise plaques full of eosinophilic material, and the tear film is grossly abnormal, very acidic and full of components of the allergic cascade. Sight is threatened even if corneal ulcerations are present transiently — if a child has an ulcer for more than a week, even once the ulcer is resolved, that child will have a certain degree of permanent loss of vision. Such patients need treatment quickly.

Patients with vernal catarrh are maintained over the winter on the mast cell stabilizers lodoxamide or nedocromil, if needed at all. Sometimes the patient does not need any treatment over this time, but in spring, when symptoms develop, mast cell stabilizers [14] together with antihistamines are required. In an acute and severe exacerbation not controlled by these agents alone, topical steroids are required, particularly if early corneal signs, such as punctuate stains, are observed. If necessary, steroids are given in up to hourly doses with dexamethasone or prednisolone, which should be preservative-free where appropriate. Hospital admission is needed if there is any question of treatment compliance or if the signs are worsening. Children usually use the eye drops, especially after one severe attack, and are often frightened enough to use the drops, even at school. Systemic therapy is not needed unless the patient also has systemic disease. The tears are abnormal, so when the eyes itch tear replacement drops, such as hypromellose, can be given which wash out the substances in the tears and stabilize the tear film. They are easy to administer and have no side-effects.

If an ulcer develops, the patient is admitted, the ulcer debrided and all of the eosinophilic material is removed. Steroids are initiated and the stromal infiltrate suppressed, so that the epithelium can slide across and reduce the risk of permanent corneal scarring. Asians, Afro-Asians and patients with severe asthma seem to have a poor prognosis and often need a large amount of systemic therapy. If patients with vernal catarrh are treated appropriately, by the time they reach puberty they will have no corneal scarring and their risk of vernal keratoconjunctivitis is reduced. However, if the disease persists and is uncontrolled, they inevitably end up with corneal scarring and long-term sight loss — but the disease generally can be controlled.

Patients with isolated eye disease usually experience a loss of 10–20% in one or both eyes. Usually only one eye is involved, but patients with co-existing atopy, particularly those in which the disease continues into adulthood, will need careful supervision.

Giant papillary conjunctivitis

Giant papillary conjunctivitis results from contact lens wear or the presence of stitches, although they are not used so frequently now except in corneal graft surgery. The pathology is probably similar to that causing vernal kerato-conjunctivitis, and the condition is treated by removing the cause. People who have atopic disease and want to wear contact lenses must keep their lenses scrupulously clean; they should wear gas-permeable lenses rather than soft contact lenses and, if necessary, they can instil a drop of lodoxamide or nedocromil before insertion and after removal of the lenses. On the whole, patients with allergic disease who have had a reaction to contact lenses should be discouraged from their use.

Future treatments

In the future, more mast cell stabilizers and antihistamines will become available. Monoclonal antibodies are in the pipeline: anti-immunoglobulin E monoclonal antibodies already have a proven effect in asthma, and anti-cytokine monoclonal antibodies on surface receptors will become available, although they seem to be effective only in specific cases. Environmental control will be helpful because if pollution falls, the number of cases is likely to fall. Allergen avoidance may extend to the use of drugs that are targeted towards the epithelium and its receptors, and so prevent the allergen entering the system.

References

1. Linneberg A, Nielsen N H, Madsen F et al. Secular trends of allergic asthma in Danish adults. The Copenhagen Allergy Study. Respir Med 2001; **95**: 258–642.

2. ISAAC. Worldwide variation in prevalence of symptoms of asthma, allergic rhinoconjunctivitis and atopic eczema. Lancet 1998: **351**: 1225–323.

3. Fleming DM, Crombie DL. Prevalence of asthma and hay fever in England and Wales. BMJ 1987; **294**: 279–83.

4. Van Eerdewegh P, Little RD, Dupuis J et al. Association of the ADAM33 gene with asthma and bronchial hyperresponsiveness. Nature 2002; **418**: 426.

5. Peat JK, Haby M, Spijker J et al. Prevalence of asthma in adults in Busselton, Western Australia. BMJ 1992; **305**: 1326–9.

6. McGill J I, Bacon A S, Anderson D et al. Allergic eye disease mechanisms — prospective article. Br J Ophthalmol 1998; **82**: 1203–14.

7. Hughes JL, Bowman-Burns C, Yeoh S-L et al. Conjunctival epithelial structure and allergic eye disease. Presented at the International Symposium on Frontiers in Ocular Immunology, Inflammation and Transplantation, London, 22–24 September 2002.

8. Wan H, Winton HL, Soeller C et al. The transmembrane protein occludin of epithelial tight junctions is a functional target for serine peptidases from faecal pellets of Dermatophagoides pteronyssinus. Clin Exp Allergy 2001; **31**: 279.

9. Schechter NM, Brass LF, Lavker RM, Jensen PJ. Reaction of mast cell proteases tryptase and chymase with protease activated receptors (PARs) on keratinocytes and fibroblasts. J Cellular Physiol 1998; **176(2)**: 365–73.

10. Davies BH, Mullins J. Topical levocabastine is more effective than Sodium Cromoglycate for the prophylaxis and treatment of seasonal allergic conjunctivitis. Allergy 1993; **48**: 519–24.

11. Ahluwalia P, Anderson DF, Wilson SJ et al. Nedocromil sodium and levocabastine reduce the symptoms of conjunctival allergen challenge by different mechanisms. JACI 2001; **108**: 449–54.

12. Van Bijsterveld OP, Kempeneers HP, Moons et al. A double-blind group comparative study of 2% nedocromil sodium and placebo in the treatment of perennial allergic conjunctivitis. Ocular Immunology and Inflammation 1994; **2**: 177–86.

13. Stokes TC, Feinburg G. Rapid onset of action of levocabastine eye-drops in histamine-induced conjunctivitis. Clin Exp Allergy 1993; **23**: 791–4.

14. Bonini S, Barney NP, Schiavone M et al. Effectiveness of nedocromil sodium 2% eye drops on clinical symptoms and tear fluid cytology of patients with vernal conjunctivitis. Eye 1992; **6**: 648–52.

Health economics of seasonal allergic conjunctivitis

Richard Wyse

This chapter considers the health economic environment surrounding the clinical effectiveness and cost effectiveness of treatments for seasonal allergic conjunctivitis in the UK. It also looks at the impact of the disease on patients' quality of life.

Decision makers in governments use health economic information to provide the evidence they need to make purchasing decisions. Pharmaceutical companies use health economics and long-term patient outcomes data to help make better decisions about their products, pricing strategies, product marketing and integration of healthcare support programmes within the NHS. With seasonal allergic conjunctivitis, resources used contribute towards short-term benefits in health (short-term symptomatic relief), long-term benefits (lifelong symptomatic relief) and limiting the severity of the disease.

Cost-effectiveness analyses

Cost effectiveness is increasingly important for all treatments because of political agendas, the national burden of disease, patient expectations and patient benefits. Many different perspectives must be taken into account when calculating the cost effectiveness of any product:

- resources consumed
- clinical outcomes
- national burden of disease
- community outcomes
- patient satisfaction with treatment
- quality of life
- health economic outcomes
- costs.

These different perspectives mean that a variety of people and organizations must be taken into account: the patient, the patient's family, the patient's employer or school, general practitioner, primary care trust, ophthalmologist, hospital manager, private health insurance providers, government and community. A number of different outcomes from the patient's point of view are considered:

- clinical outcomes (signs and symptoms, scientific evaluation, morbidity and adverse events)
- patient satisfaction (quality and success of treatment, convenience of treatment and ability and willingness to pay)
- patient quality of life (physical function, social integration and ability to work and/or perform desired tasks)
- economic outcomes (cost of procedures, tests, drugs, physician, ophthalmologist and nurse time, and time off work – losses to employers and employees).

A cost effective analysis involves an examination of the cash flow involved in managing the patient population over a few months of the year with a choice of treatments. A number of different types of evaluations exist:

- cost analysis
- cost–minimization analysis
- cost–effectiveness analysis
- cost–utility analysis
- cost–benefit analysis
- burden of disease study
- cost of illness study.

Some of these methodologies have been directed at allergic conjunctivitis. Cost–effectiveness analyses are able to compare treatments that are not equally effective — provided there is a common though not necessarily identical outcome, different alternatives can be compared using money as the common unit. Such analyses are reported in terms of, for example, 'cost per millimetre drop in blood pressure' or 'cost per successful case'. Some published work of this type involves seasonal allergic conjunctivitis. Cost–utility analyses compare treatments that differ in the way they affect quality of life, for example surgery versus drugs or perhaps dietary supplementation. This allows the analyst to introduce quality of life information, such as sickness impact profiles, short form-36 results and ocular specific questionnaires, into a cost effective analysis.

A burden of disease study would be able to show the impact of seasonal allergic conjunctivitis for the country and would involve an analysis of all the direct and indirect costs associated with the condition — everything needed to manage the patients. No such UK study has been reported to date.

Health economics cannot demonstrate better cost-effectiveness of any treatment without some measurable improvements in efficacy or a better safety profile. This means that positive clinical benefits must be demonstrated before positive financial benefits can be calculated or cost-effectiveness shown.

Some analyses have attempted to put a value on quality of life. For example, patients experiencing poor vision due to macular degeneration would trade between two and six years of perfect vision for every 10 years of remaining life [1, 2]. These data have some relevance for seasonal allergic conjunctivitis, even though this condition is not life- or sight-threatening.

Impact of seasonal allergic conjunctivitis in the UK

Seasonal allergic conjunctivitis presents an important public health problem. It has a high incidence in the UK population and presents a large national burden. The condition is recurrent, so every year it causes substantial discomfort and greatly affects patients' daily work, school and social lives.

The substantial costs of care are supported by the UK's health budget, and numerous purchases of over-the-counter therapies are also involved in treatment of the disease in the UK. Health economic analyses must take into account issues of efficacy of therapy, cost effectiveness, rate of onset, comfort of therapy, safety of therapy (including the cost of adverse events), topical versus systemic therapy, drowsiness, creation of dry eye, risk of adverse drug interactions with co-medications and patient satisfaction with treatment. They must also take into account patients' ability and willingness to pay: if a patient must wait for an appointment with their general practitioner, they are likely to go and purchase their own medications over the counter.

In the UK, allergic conjunctivitis represents a leading cause of acute red eye presentation to both hospital and general practitioners [3]. Seasonal allergic conjunctivitis is thought to affect around 10% of the UK population [4], although the UK prevalence based on patients seen at a health centre in three summer months was estimated as 21% [3]. A number of different studies offer different values, but local variation is common: for example, prevalence of itchy eye in North Thames is 15.9% whereas in Scotland it is 20.3% [5].

The symptoms of seasonal allergic conjunctivitis affect patients' quality of life. The disease results in visits to the general practitioner, lost productivity at work, impact on employer, loss of time at school, social life restrictions and compromise of vision-related activities. Approximately 75% of people with seasonal allergic conjunctivitis who also wear contact lenses report very significant discomfort [6]. A study by Dart et al collated a quality of life score with seven components: itchiness, photophobia, redness, grittiness, epiphora, mucus discharge and swelling [7]. Each component was scored from 0 (no effect on quality of life) to 4 (major effect), with the maximum possible score of 28 corresponding to the worst quality of life. The mean score per eye was 9.3 for seasonal allergic conjunctivitis compared with 1.1 for perennial allergic conjunctivitis; this proves the relative severity of the symptoms of seasonal allergic conjunctivitis.

Cost effectiveness

As an example of a cost–effectiveness study, a recent and highly detailed investigation by Claude Le Pen reported a method to derive an aggregated symptom score for assessing treatment efficacy in seasonal allergic conjunctivitis. The aggregated symptom score was calculated using a weighted system, which brought together and synthesized into a single measurable parameter, the relative severities of all the diverse major ocular and nasal symptoms experienced by each patient whilst suffering from seasonal allergic conjunctivitis [8]. The first stage was a comparison of efficacy. The authors plotted mean ocular scores for olopatadine versus levocabastine from day 0 to day 42 for itching, redness, eyelid swelling and physician's impression of the treatment. Although both drugs work very well, olopatadine seemed to be favoured statistically and the authors concluded that olopatadine was consistently better than levocabastine in improving secondary signs and in physicians' impression.

Once a measurable improvement in efficacy was shown for olopatadine, the same authors performed a cost–effectiveness analysis in six countries: France, Germany, Italy, Spain, Sweden and the UK (Le Pen, unpublished data). They developed a cost:effective ratio called 'cost per symptoms adjusted days', which represented the number of days wasted by the severity of symptoms, and a cost:utility ratio, termed 'quality adjusted days'. The cost of care was determined through analysis of a questionnaire that surveyed the type and number of laboratory tests and examinations or procedures usually prescribed to patients with seasonal allergic conjunctivitis, the frequency of visits to the doctor (ophthalmologists, general practitioners and/or other specialists) and the standard treatment given to patients with seasonal allergic conjunctivitis (with precision about the daily dose, form and duration of treatment in days). Experts distinguished between the three levels of severity of symptoms (low, moderate and severe), because they are likely to have an impact on medical resource usage.

Costs relating to general practitioners', ophthalmologists' and allergologists' consultations were determined by applying a unit cost to the number of consultations or visits recorded in the trial. National differences were taken into account: in Germany and Spain, for instance, the first consultation is more expensive than subsequent consultations, while in the UK, general practitioner consultations were not valued because general practitioners are paid under a capitation system. This means that the results of the study are comprehensive for the other five countries, but not so for the UK.

Juniper et al had previously developed 28- and 14-item questionnaires about quality of life in patients with rhinoconjunctivitis and reported that the questionnaires had strong evaluative and discriminative properties over and above the short form-36 [9, 10]. In fact, measuring symptom severity in a single dimension is not necessarily representative of the impact on patient quality of life. Transformation from a symptom score to a quality of life score may be needed. The Le Pen study attempts to correlate utility with symptoms and produces a mathematical analysis of the data, which in turn produces good health economic arguments (Le Pen, unpublished data). Because of the different (GP gatekeeper) healthcare system used in the UK, the necessary exclusion of general practitioner consultations from the analysis of trial data means that the results from the UK are very different from those of the other countries (Figure 1). Unfortunately these results can therefore not be fully

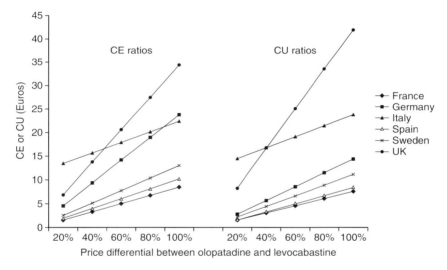

FIGURE 1 Cost–effectiveness (CE) analysis and cost–utility (CU) analysis of olopatadine versus levocabastine (Le Pen, unpublished data)

The CE ratio is the 'cost per symptoms adjusted days' (which represents the number of days weighted by the level of severity of symptoms). The CU ratio represents quality-adjusted days. At the two right-hand price differential points, the UK data can be readily identified by the uppermost CE line (reaching 35 Euros) and the uppermost CU line (reaching 42 Euros)

relied on. However, analyses of the type shown in Figure 1 allow healthcare purchasers and providers a rational analysis of which medication would be the most cost-effective to purchase in a particular context. These analyses allow a transparent purchasing choice between two medications by balancing their difference in price against their difference in efficacy. Overall, even given the superior efficacy of olopatadine, Figure 1 shows a 20–60% higher price compared to that of levocabastine is justifiable in several European countries, both in terms of the number of symptom-free days and improvements in patient quality of life.

Other studies

In a national burden of disease study, Ray *et al* estimated the cost to the USA of allergic rhinoconjunctivitis at $1.9 billion as a primary diagnosis and $4 billion as a secondary diagnosis [11]. Of this total $5.9 billion, outpatient services comprised $3.7 billion, drugs $1.5 billion and inpatient services $0.7 billion. The USA has approximately five times the population of the UK.

The study by Katelaris *et al* emphasized the impact of the negative effects of seasonal allergic conjunctivitis on quality of life and athletic performance in a series of olympic and para-olympic athletes [12]. Cakmak *et al* found that there was a 10% statistically significant increase in emergency visits to a children's hospital for conjunctivitis and rhinitis once specific airborne pollens and spores exceeded certain concentrations [13].

Summary

Treatments for seasonal allergic conjunctivitis impact on patient quality of life and the patient's ability to work. Available therapeutic options differ in their efficacy, time course and cost. Whilst relatively new to the UK, there is a wealth of clinical experience in the USA on the effective use of olopatadine to treat seasonal allergic conjunctivitis. Of the small amount of clinical and health economic studies conducted in seasonal allergic conjunctivitis in the UK and Europe, it would appear that the use of olopatadine may confer cost-effective advantages to healthcare purchasers, both in terms of the reduced number of pateint days affected versus the severity of their symptoms on these days, and also from the perspective of improvements in patient quality of life-adjusted days.

References

1. Brown GC, Brown MM, Sharma S. Difference between ophthalmologists' and patients' perceptions of quality of life associated with age-related macular degeneration. *Can J Ophthalmol* 2000; **35**: 127–33.

2. Brown GC. Vision and quality of life. *Trans Am Ophthalmol Soc* 1999; 97: 473–511.

3. Dart JKG. Eye disease at a community health centre. *BMJ* 1986; **293**: 1477–80.

4. Davies BH, Mullins J. Topical levocabastine is more effective than sodium cromoglycate for the prophylaxis and treatment of seasonal allergic conjunctivitis. *Allergy* 1993; **48**: 519–24.

5. Strachan D, Sibbald B, Weiland S *et al*. Worldwide variations in prevalence of symptoms of allergic rhinoconjunctivitis in children: the International Study of Asthma and Allergies in Childhood (ISAAC). *Pediatr Allergy Immunol* 1997; **8(4)**: 161–76.

6. Kumar P, Erstol R, Black D. Allergic rhinoconjunctivitis and contact lens intolerance. *CLAO J* 1991; **17(1)**: 31–4.

7. Dart JK, Buckley RJ, Monnickendan M, Prasad J. Perennial allergic conjunctivitis: definition, clinical

characteristics and prevalence. A comparison with seasonal allergic conjunctivitis. *Trans Ophthamol Soc UK* 1986; **105**: 513–20.

8. Le Pen C, Smith AF, Lilliu H, Priol G. A method to derive an aggregated score for assessing treatment efficacy in seasonal allergic conjunctivitis. *Clinical Drug Invest* 2002; **22**: 783–9.

9. Juniper EF, Thompson AK, Ferrie PJ, Roberts JN. Development and validation of the mini Rhinoconjunctivitis Quality of Life Questionnaire. *Clin Exp Allergy* 2000; **30**: 132–40.

10. Juniper EF, Thompson AK, Roberts JN. Can the standard gamble and rating scale be used to measure quality of life in rhinoconjunctivitis? Comparison with the RQLQ and SF-36. *Allergy* 2002; **57**: 201–6.

11. Ray NF, Baraniuk JN, Thamer M *et al.* Direct expenditures for the treatment of allergic rhinoconjunctivitis in 1996, including the contributions of related airway illnesses. *J Allergy Clin Immunol* 1999; **103**: 401–7.

12. Katelaris CH, Carrozzi FM, Burke TV, Byth K. Effects of intranasal budesonide on symptoms, quality of life, and performance in elite athletes with allergic rhinoconjunctivitis. *Clin J Sport Med* 2002; **12**: 296–300.

13. Cakmak S, Dales RE, Burnett RT *et al.* Effect of airborne allergens on emergency visits by children for conjunctivitis and rhinitis. *Lancet* 2002; **359**: 947–8.

Discussion

MARK ABELSON: In the quality of life score by Dart that you described [1], the included symptoms — grittiness, swelling, mucous discharge, redness and photophobia — could equally well, or perhaps better, define conditions other than seasonal allergic conjunctivitis. It does not seem realistic to think that seasonal allergic conjunctivitis is 10 times as serious as perennial allergic conjunctivitis.

DERMOT RYAN: That is a symptom score rather than a quality of life score. A paper by John Bousquet [2] compares quality of life in seasonal allergic rhinoconjunctivitis and asthma and shows that seasonal allergic rhinoconjunctivitis gives a worse quality of life than people suffering from asthma.

MARK ABELSON: We use a quality of life questionnaire in our group that has been used in a 400–500 patient study. It is a modification and improvement upon Juniper's study, which only has quality of life for rhinoconjunctivitis [3], and does not mention much about the eyes. I think the study you discussed extrapolating symptomatology and signs to quality of life is flawed. If my eye burns for 5 minutes, how much effect on quality of life is that? Would I trade two years of my life for an extra two years of poor vision?

RICHARD WYSE: I think your argument works well for cataracts. It also works for macular degeneration especially in view of the inadequate treatment for this disease. In seasonal allergic conjunctivitis, there is a treatment. I was not part of that study [1], but it is the best study that I've seen in Europe — very few studies have been published in this field.

DERMOT RYAN: I do not understand the need for a study like this. A new drug coming into this market has to show itself to be at least as effective as existing preparations and to be easier to use, more preferred by patients and effective at keeping patients out of the surgery. The bottom line is that the product needs to come in below the market leader on price and to show it is a better drug.

MARK ABELSON: Are these data a requirement of the European Union or of a specific government or are they pharmaceutical industry data?

RICHARD WYSE: We have a National Institute of Clinical Excellence that can request and act upon this information.

DERMOT RYAN: General practitioners just want simple information about efficacy and patient preference; price sensitivity comes lower down in the list of priorities.

References

1. Dart JK, Buckley RJ, Monnickendan M, Prasad J. Perennial allergic conjunctivitis: definition, clinical characteristics and prevalence. A comparison with seasonal allergic conjunctivitis. *Trans Ophthalmol Soc UK* 1986; **105**: 513–20.

2. Leynaert B, Neukirch C, Liard R et al. Quality of life in allergic rhinitis and asthma: A population-based study of young adults. *Am J Respir Crit Care Med* 2000; **162**: 1391–6.

3. Juniper EF, Thompson AK, Ferrie PJ, Roberts JN. Development and validation of the mini Rhinoconjunctivitis Quality of Life Questionnaire. *Clin Exp Allergy* 2000; **57**: 201–6.

The American perspective — clinical experience of a new treatment

Mark Abelson

The estimated point prevalence of seasonal allergic conjunctivitis is 20% of the general population — over 50 million people in the USA [1]. Most people develop allergies in childhood, but a small group develops post-pubescent allergy between the ages of 18 and 35 years. Patients present to their general practitioner complaining of itchy, red, swollen eyes and sometimes a splitting headache.

Mast cells

The eyes contain many mast cells — more are located nasally rather than temporally. In the quiescent eye, the mast cells are found in the substantia propra. In patients with a severe and/or chronic allergic reaction, the number of mast cells increases and they tend to be found in more superficial parts of the eye.

Mast cells are a heterogeneous group and are species- and tissue-specific [2]. The various types of mast cells fall into two main categories:

- tryptase-containing human mast cells, which are found in the mucosa
- tryptase/chymase-containing cells, which are found in the connective tissue and conjunctiva.

Different types of mast cells respond differently to different drugs, so some drugs may be effective in the respiratory passages and some on the ocular surface. For example, tryptase-containing cells respond to doxantrazole and quercetin, while tryptase/chymase-containing cells respond to both of these agents, as well as to disodium cromoglycate and theophylline [3]. In one study, cromolyn, nedocromil and pemirolast all failed significantly to inhibit histamine release from human conjunctival mast cells stimulated with immunoglobulin (Ig) E, while olopatadine produced a significant concentration-dependent inhibition of histamine release [4].

Mast cells are often considered to be most active in ocular allergy, but their major function is homeostasis and control of the microvasculature, which they achieve by dilatation and contraction of the microvascular networks throughout the body by way of release of vasoactive amines. In addition, given their known role in wound healing in other parts of the body, such as the skin, they are currently being looked at as also having a role in wound healing in the eye by releasing their contents into the tear film. The process of mast cell degranulation in allergy involves the following steps:

- allergen crosslinks specific IgE
- calcium ions pour into the mast cell's cytoplasm
- microtubules lead granules to the cell membrane
- the contents of the mast cell are released into the extracellular space; this includes histamine, tryptase, chymase, heparin, cytokines, chemokines, vasoactive peptides, prostaglandin D_2, interleukin-1 (IL-1), IL-4, tumour necrosis factor-α (TNF-α), intercellular adhesion molecule-1 (ICAM-1), eotaxin, leukotriene C_4 and platelet-activating factor
- the calcium also helps to mediate the activation of phospholipase and the breakdown of aracidonic acid into prostaglandins and leukotrienes.

Histamine

Histamine is the primary mediator of allergic conjunctivitis. Two histamine receptors have been identified on the ocular surface; stimulation of H_1 on nerve endings produces itching while stimulation of H_1 and H_2 receptors on blood vessels leads to vasodilatation (evident as redness) and endothelial gaping and leakage of fluid from the vessel into the surrounding tissue, producing lid swelling and chemosis. [5].

Histamine causes itching, redness and swelling in a dose-dependent fashion [6]. In patients with vernal conjunctivitis, levels of histamine are very high. Histamine is very important in seasonal allergic conjunctivitis, but it is not the only mediator: histamine-induced itching and vasodilatation in the skin can be enhanced by mixing histamine with prostaglandin D_2 [7]. Histamine is an excellent marker for seasonal and perennial allergic conjunctivitis and might be considered to be pathognomonic.

By adding pollen to the eyes of people with seasonal allergic conjunctivitis, release of histamine can be stimulated [8]. In one study, histamine was instilled into human eyes [6]. Itching peaked at three minutes, before reducing because of the action of histaminase. Redness and chemosis both peaked at 20 minutes.

Instillation of a secretagogue (compound 48/80) into the eyes of animals and humans induced degranulation of mast cells, released histamine and induced allergic conjunctivitis [9]. This study was interesting in that a similar pattern of response was seen whether the allergic response was induced with histamine, the secretagogue or pollen.

In patients with vernal conjunctivitis, itching is relentless; in patients with seasonal allergic conjunctivitis, itching is self-limited. This difference is explained by a deficiency of histaminase in patients with vernal conjunctivitis, which causes histamine levels to remain very high for long periods. In seasonal allergic conjunctivitis histamine is difficult to recover from the eye because it is quickly degraded by normally functioning histaminase. If tear samples are treated with histaminase inactivator, histamine can be recovered from the eye in seasonal allergic conjunctivitis [10]. Histamine levels are shown to peak at three minutes after challenge in seasonal allergic conjunctivitis [11]. This shows that histamine is bioavailable in tears very soon after challenge — before it binds to the histamine receptors or is cleaved by histaminases, eg histidine decarboxylase, into its breakdown products.

Ocular effects of histamine

Lid swelling occurs as a result of vasodilatation of blood vessels. The fact that the conjunctiva is bound down to the tarsal plate and that the tissue in the lid is extremely weak provides the perfect circumstances for leaky vessels, produced by H_1- or H_2-induced gaping, to lead to lid swelling and chemosis. There is also a propensity towards residual lid swelling the next morning.

The late phase phenomenon, which is the secondary occurrence of symptomatology and signs six hours after antigen challenge, only seems to occur in 1–2% of cases of seasonal allergic conjunctivitis, but it does occur in vernal, atopic and perennial conjunctivitis. In tear studies in patients with seasonal allergic conjunctivitis, increases were seen in the number of neutrophils, eosinophils and lymphocytes present in tears at six hours [12]. A small increase in levels of ICAM-1 shows that increases occur not only in the number of cells, but also in the number of sites available for their adherence. In 99% of cases, this effect is below the threshold for producing symptoms and patients do not have any increased swelling, itching or redness at the six-hour time point [13].

Differential diagnoses

Non-specific conjunctivitis is an issue during differential diagnosis because many doctors tend to group together patients with itching eyes and those with burning eyes. In reality, the patients with burning symptoms have dry eye conditions and those with itching have allergic disease.

Drug-induced conjunctivitis disproportionately affects the lower parts of the lid. It produces prominent redness and chemosis, which is followed by chronic chemosis and dermatitis inferiorly. This results in a vicious circle because the patient pulls and holds down the lower lid with their finger and applies the drops in to the cul-de-sac, then the drops spill over on to the lower lid. The condition is relentlessly progressive, and the longer the patient takes the drops, the worse it gets.

As we saw earlier, 20% of the population have allergy [1]. About 6–7% of the population have dry eye at any one time [14, 15], but almost all of the population at some point will have a dry eye condition, perhaps caused by aeroplane travel, sitting near a hot fan or in a heated car, working with a computer, performing prolonged visual tasks like reading or using a systemic antihistaminic drug. In such patients, a tear substitute and guidance on avoiding possible causes is sufficient to relieve the redness, irritation and grittiness.

The most important diagnostic clues are:

- If it itches, it is allergy.
- If it burns, it is dry eye.
- If it's sticky, it is bacterial conjunctivitis.

Colour is another important indicator for diagnosis. Fire engine red indicates deep scleritis, endopthalmitis, anterior segment ischaemia or a corneal ulcer. Pink suggests a less serious condition — perhaps seasonal allergic conjunctivitis or a quandrantic marginal infiltrate.

Quality of life

Allergy has a significant impact on patients' quality of life. It affects their sleep, productivity (whether at work or school), social interactions and their ability to perform visual tasks. It also has cosmetic implications because of the lid swelling, redness and tearing.

In many instances, the patient is better able to diagnose their allergic conjunctivitis than their doctor. Doctors rarely ask about allergies out of the pollen season and in the USA, 90% of patients with seasonal allergic conjunctivitis treat themselves with over-the-counter medications— once they get symptoms, they do not want to wait for an appointment. By integrating questions about allergies in to the general history and asking patients (even when seeing them in the off-season) if their eyes itch at times, physicians will uncover more patients with allergies who can benefit from a more effective treatment than the over-the-counter agents that most patients use.

Treatment options

Non-pharmacological treatment options include tear substitutes, cold compresses and avoidance of allergen sources. Tear substitutes serve a number of purposes in allergic conjunctivitis. They provide a barrier across the entry point for pollen and they can reduce the concentrations of allergens and mediators in the tears or flush them out of the eyes.

In the USA, pharmacological management includes:

- antihistamines
- antihistamine/vasoconstrictor combinations

- mast cell stabilizers
- antihistamine/mast cell stabilizers
- steroids
- immunomodulators.

Antihistamines

The H_1-antihistamines successfully relieve the itch of allergy, but fail to inhibit other histamine receptor subtypes and other pro-inflammatory mediators such as prostaglandins and leukotrienes. Levocabastine and emedastine are the topical antihistamines available in the USA as prescription eye drops. They have a rapid onset of action, but they only provide short-term symptomatic relief [16]. Emedastine is more potent and has a longer duration of action (about four hours) [17].

Antihistamine/vasoconstrictor combinations

Vasoconstrictors are sympathomimetic adrenergic agents that reduce infection and swelling. Antihistamine/vasoconstrictor combinations block the effects of histamines to prevent itching, while producing vasoconstriction to reduce redness. They can only be used four times a day and they last for just under two hours, which leaves the patient unprotected for about half a day. The vasoconstrictors used in such combinations — eg naphazoline — are notoriously tachyphylactic and have the potential for causing paediatric problems when overused.

Mast cell stabilizers

The exact mechanism of the mast cell stabilizers is unclear, but they may:

- inhibit influx of calcium ions into the cell after the antigen binds
- affect membrane fluidity
- inhibit phosphorylation of necessary proteins.

It is clear, however, that mast cell stabilizers prevent the production of newly formed mediators and also prevent mast cell degranulation by inhibiting the release of pre-formed mediators such as histamine and chemotactic factors [18]. The available agents are nedocromil, pemirolast, lodoxamide and cromolyn. In vernal conjunctivitis, lodoxamide is particularly effective at reducing keratitis but the amount of redness, swelling and itching was not consistently different between patients who were treated with lodoxamide and those who were untreated [19].

The biggest difference was seen in the amount of keratitis and the number of vernal ulcers between the groups. This suggested that Iodoxamide had a direct effect on eosinophils. It may act on one of the proteases released during mast cell granulation, but it seems unlikely that Iodoxamide is a mast cell stabilizer, although it works very effectively as a protector of the ocular surface.

Antihistamine/mast cell stabilizers

The antihistamine/mast cell stabilizers include olopatadine, ketotifen and azelastine. Azelastine was investigated in 1980 as a potential therapy, but it was not comfortable in the eye and the work was stopped. It is a H_1-antihistamine and has been considered as a mast cell stabilizer because it produces anti-inflammatory effects [20]. Of note however is that this work was not done in human conjunctival mast cells. Ketotifen is a very potent agent for itching, but at the concentration at which it works best, it is uncomfortable in the eye [21]. Olopatadine is indicated for all the signs and symptoms of allergic conjunctivitis (itching, redness, tearing and chemosis) and is very comfortable in the eye [22].

Agents with multiple modes of activity offer significant advantages in that they can prevent an ongoing reaction effectively with the antihistamine component, but also work to keep all the mediators in the mast cell, which helps their duration of action.

Steroids

Steroids cross cell membranes to bind to receptors in the cytosol. The steroid–receptor complex is transported to the nucleus where it affects protein metabolism. This inhibits production of prostaglandins and leukotrienes, as well as cytokine and adhesion molecule formation. Side-effects include delayed wound healing, secondary infections, elevated intraocular pressure and cataract formation, so treatment should be monitored by an eye-care professional. Steroids should only be used in chronic, severe cases of ocular allergy and those that do not respond to other drugs. It also can be seen simply from their mechanism of action and the pathophysiology of the allergic reaction how they are not helpful in an acute setting.

Immunomodulators

Immunomodulators are another treatment option because of their T-cell suppression. Time will tell if this class has a therapeutic role in seasonal allergies. By the nature of their mechanisms, they would probably be useful for chronic severe cases. Tacrolimus is available for dermatitis and could be used for dermatitis of the lids in acute keratoconjunctivitis.

Topical versus systemic therapy

It is important to treat topical diseases topically for a number of reasons. Topical drugs provide direct delivery to the desired site and higher concentrations at the target, and they are not prone to interactions with alcohol or central nervous system depressants. By comparison, systemically administered agents have more side-effects (eg sedation, dizziness, tinnitus, nervousness and insomnia).

Another consideration is that although systemic antihistamines are non-sedating they are not non-drying. A study examined the effects of loratadine on tear flow and volume [23]. Fluorophotometry was used to measure tear flow and volume before and after four days of dosing with loratadine. After dosing with loratadine for four days in a dose-dependent fashion, patients were less tolerant of adverse environmental conditions, with increased ocular discomfort scores and increased keratitis. Similar results were found with terfenadine and cetirizine. This is due to the antihistamines' anti-muscarinic action. Because of this, the tear film's ability to protect the eye is diminished. Tears are important as a barrier function, diluent and eyewash. By decreasing these effects, allergens can more easily penetrate on to the ocular surface to stimulate mast cells, and the tear film will not be as effective in washing the mediators away. Oral antihistamines have no place in treating eye allergy. If there is any ocular component (indicated by any ocular itching), a topical ocular treatment should be used. In fact, in patients who also have nasal allergies, eye drops will give added effect to nasal therapy in treating the nasal symptoms by the nature of their drainage from the eye to the nose.

Research models

The standard antigen challenge model involves four patient visits. At visit one, the threshold to reactivity is determined. At visit two, the patient's allergy status is confirmed and if redness or itching scores are lower than 2 on the 0–4 scale [8], they are excluded. Visit three is used to determine the drug's speed of onset: the test drug or placebo is administered and the patient is challenged 10–15 minutes later and evaluated. Visit four determines the drug's duration of action: the drug or placebo is administered and the patient is challenged eight hours after challenge and evaluated.

In this model, the patient is challenged before they are started on the drug for a period of up to several months to ensure that they are responsive. This model assumes that patients are significantly responsive to pollen in season and allows the effects of repetitive usage over the entire season to be determined.

Development of olopatadine

Olopatadine was first conceived in the mid 1990s. Some agents were noted to act in the lab as combined mast cell stabilizers and antihistamines, but none were available in the clinic — all were still being tested in rats. Dr John Yanni screened these compounds and found that one particular molecule, olopatadine, seemed to respond to human conjunctival mast cell explants [24].

Olopatadine was successfully launched in the USA four years ago. It currently accounts for 65% of the US market for anti-allergic drugs, and it more than tripled the size of the antiallergic market from about $70 million to over $300 million in 2002. It is used solely in ophthalmology and was the first drug developed because of its effects on human conjunctival mast cells. It is currently not available for systemic, nasal or oral use.

Olopatadine works on multiple targets: it is a potent antihistamine and a potent mast cell stabilizer that inhibits the release of histamine, IL-4, TNF-α and eotaxin. It has anti-inflammatory properties and decreases the regulation of anti-immunoglobulin E mast cell-mediated upregulation of ICAM-1 [25–28]. Pre-treatment with olopatadine before conjunctival allergen challenge resulted in lower tear levels of histamine than with placebo (7 versus 22.4 nm/l), as well as lower cellular infiltrates and ICAM expression. The expected peak of histamine concentration at 3–5 minutes was greatly reduced with such treatment, and clearly demonstrating that olopatadine is working as a mast cell stabilizer. Irkec looked at the effects of olopatadine on eotaxin and found that olopatadine dramatically reduced its release in allergic patients [29]. Such evidence confirms that olopatadine is a dual-action agent. It has been approved in the USA for the treatment of all of the signs and symptoms of seasonal allergic conjunctivitis (itching, redness, chemosis, tearing, mucous damage and lid swelling). The mast cell-stabilizing activity helps olopatadine to prevent the release of histamine, vasoactive peptides, chemokines, cytokines and other mediators from the mast cell.

Clinical trials

Multiple studies compared the effects of olopatadine against placebo in the treatment of allergic conjunctivitis; all showed that olopatadine reduced vasodilatation, gaping and swelling, as well as chemosis [30]. In one environmental study in which patients with allergic conjunctivitis or allergic rhinoconjunctivitis were dosed with either olopatadine or placebo during the allergy season, both itching and redness were reduced. Of note is that nasal symptoms were also reduced. This is because eye drops drain out of the eye through the nasolacrimal duct and into the inferior turbinate where the drug can also exert its activity. As a drug can drain to the nose, so can mediators. Thus a drug such as olopatadine that can prevent the mast cell from degranulating will reduce the number of mediators that drain and produce symptoms in the nose.

Olopatadine has been studied extensively and compared with many other agents in double-blind, placebo-controlled studies. The clinical efficacy of olopatadine and nedocromil were compared in the human conjunctival allergen challenge model [31]. Between visits two and three, subjects instilled nedocromil in one eye and placebo in the contralateral eye twice-daily for two weeks. At visit three, before antigen challenge, participants received one drop of olopatadine in the eye dosed with placebo and one drop of nedocromil in the eye dosed with nedocromil for the previous two weeks. Eyes treated with one drop of olopatadine had statistically significant reductions of itching compared with eyes treated with 29 drops of nedocromil (Figure 1). Patient ratings of the eye drop comfort were statistically significant in favour of olopatadine over nedocromil: in the 17 patients who received olopatadine in one eye and nedocromil in the other eye, 14 (71%)

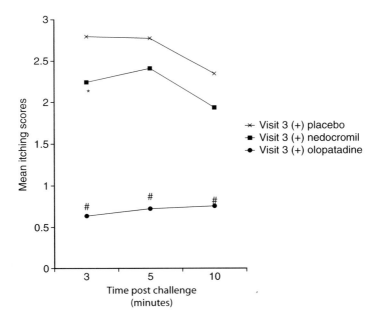

FIGURE 1   Comparison of onset of action for olopatadine, nedocromil and placebo. #$p<0.05$ between olopatadine and both nedocromil- and placebo-treated eyes; *$p<0.05$ between nedocromil- and placebo-treated eyes

patients preferred olopatadine, 3 (29%) expressed no preference and none preferred nedocromil.

Olopatadine was successfully compared with ketotifen [21, 22, 32] and azelastine, the two other drugs in its c ass.

The efficacy of olopatadine was compared with that of azelastine in the conjunctival allergen challenge model [33]. Every minute, from five minutes after treatment with the test drug, the patient was asked whether their eyes itched. This allowed the production of a curve to show the pattern and time course of itching. The results show that olopatadine reduces itching more than azelastine throughout the entire time course of itching. Another study compared the comfort of olopatadine with that of azelastine [34]. The top three descriptive words used by participants immediately after instillation of drops were moisturizing, comfortable and refreshing for olopatadine and stinging, burning and irritating for azelastine. Overall, 68 (72.5%) participants preferred olopatadine compared with 13 (14.5%) who preferred azelastine; the remainder had no preference. These results showed that olopatadine was more effective than azelastine in managing itch associated with allergic conjunctivitis and was significantly more comfortable.

Steroids should be reserved for severe chronic cases of allergy; in these cases loteprednol is the steroid of choice as it is the only steroid approved in the USA for allergic conjunctivitis. The clinical efficacy and safety of olopatadine was compared with loteprednol in patients with acute seasonal allergic conjunctivitis [35]. Fifty patients with a history of allergic conjunctivitis were randomized to receive olopatadine, loteprednol or placebo (ratio 2:2:1). Loteprednol requires a loading period to achieve maximum efficacy, so patients assigned this treatment received loteprednol four times daily bilaterally for a 14-day period. Patients in the olopatadine and placebo groups received placebo four times daily in each eye for this loading period. Mean redness and itching scores showed that one drop of olopatadine was more efficacious than a two-week loading period with loteprednol in reducing the itching and redness associated with seasonal allergic conjunctivitis (Figure 2). With respect to intraocular pressure, a statistically significant increase was seen with loteprednol but not with placebo or olopatadine.

The onset of action of olopatadine instilled in the eye was compared with that of oral loratadine by obtaining itching scores in the antigen challenge model two and eight hours after dosing [36]. The results showed that olopatadine was significantly more efficacious than loratadine at reducing ocular itching associated with allergic conjunctivitis and, when used in combination, improved the effect of loratadine.

The safety and efficacy of the concomitant use of fluticasone nasal spray and olopatadine eye drops were compared with those of concomitant use of oral fexofenadine and fluticasone nasal spray and placebo eye drops in subjects with allergic rhinoconjunctivitis in the conjunctival allergen challenge model [37]. Between visits two and three, decreases in ocular itching scores for olopatadine and

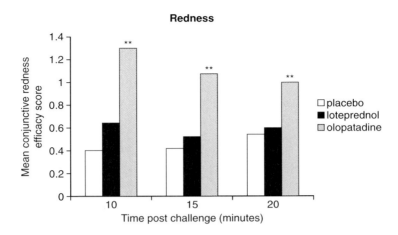

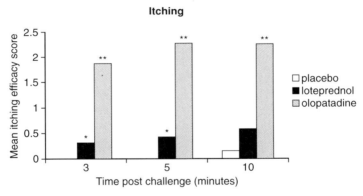

FIGURE 2 Mean conjunctival redness and itching efficacy scores with olopatadine, loteprednol and placebo

0 → 2.5 on mean efficacy score is from low → higher efficacy

fluticasone were statistically significant compared with those of fexofenadine and fluticasone. Concomitant use of olopatadine and fluticasone was superior to use of fluticasone and fexofenadine combination therapy for overall treatment of the signs and symptoms of allergic rhinoconjunctivitis. This study shows that when patients with rhinoconjunctivitis present with nasal and ocular components, control is best achieved using an eye drop and a nasal spray together.

Comfort of olopatadine in the treatment of allergic conjunctivitis in contact lens wearers was compared with that of placebo in the conjunctival allergen challenge model [38]. Statistically significant differences in comfort were observed at one- to 10-minute time-points ($p < 0.05$). Clinically significant superiority was noted at the additional time points of 15 through 30 minutes (>1 unit difference). Patients that received olopatadine showed a clinically significant difference in duration of contact lens wear from time of insertion at study visit to time of removal by subject after leaving study visit, with lens wearers averaging 2.1 hours longer than those who received placebo. The results show that olopatadine was clinically and significantly superior to placebo in improving the ocular comfort of contact lens wearers. Olopatadine also allowed for longer duration of lens wear than placebo.

Summary

The use of agents that have both antihistamine and mast cell-stabilizing properties has significant advantages. Because histamine is the primary mediator in eye allergy, a potent blocker of histamine receptors on nerve endings and blood vessels is important. The mast cell-stabilizing component helps to keep other mediators from being released, and it gives the agent preventive ability and longer duration of action. However, as considerable mast cell heterogeneity exists between tissues and between species, it is important that mast cell-stabilizing effects for eye allergy are evaluated in human conjunctival mast cells. Of note are several studies in cell cultures and in humans that demonstrate the effective mast cell-stabilizing activity of olopatadine. Further, olopatadine is the only drug in its class indicated not only for itching, but also for all the signs and symptoms of allergic conjunctivitis — direct evidence that olopatadine has clinically relevant mast cell-stabilizing properties.

By blocking the release of mediators other than histamine, eg vasoactive peptides, from the mast cell, olopatadine can be expected to have significant effects on swelling as well. This is specifically of importance as redness and swelling have important quality of life and cosmetic implications. The mast cell-stabilizing activity may also play a future role in regulating wound healing, as mast cell mediators can be expected to be released into the tear film during corneal healing.

In numerous studies, olopatadine has been compared and shown to be superior to each of the other drugs and other classes used to treat ocular allergy. Of note is that a single drop of olopatadine is more effective than a two-week loading period of either a mast cell-stabilizer or steroid. Compliance with olopatadine is aided by its comfort.

Often patients will present with nasal symptoms as well as eye symptoms. In these cases, treatment with topical therapy is best. From a pharmacokinetic point of view systemic antihistamines cannot deliver as much drug to the eye, and they also have significant drying effects on the ocular surface. Systemic antihistamines have no role in treating patients who have an ocular component. The ideal therapy for patients with allergic rhinoconjunctivitis is a potent allergy eye drop and a nasal spray. In fact, remember that treating the eye with an eye drop will also help relieve nasal symptoms by preventing mediators draining from the eye into the nose and by the drug itself draining into the nose.

References

1. Dart JK, Buckley RJ, Monnickendam M, Prasad J. Perennial allergic conjunctivitis: definition, clinical characteristics and prevalence. Trans Ophthalmol Soc UK 1986; **105**: 513–20.

2. Irani AA, Schwartz LB. Human mast cell heterogeneity. Allergy Proc 1994; **15(6)**: 303–8.

3. Abelson MB. Allergic diseases of the eye. Philadelphia: W B Saunders Company, 2001; p24.

4. Yanni JM, Miller ST, Garnache DA et al. Comparative effects of topical ocular anti-allergy drugs on human conjunctival mast cells. Ann Allergy Asthma Immunol 1997; **79(6)**: 541–5.

5. Abelson MB, Udell IJ. H$_2$-receptors in the human ocular surface. Arch Ophthalmology 1981; **99**: 302–4.

6. Abelson MB, Allansmith MR. Immunology and immunopathology of the eye. New York: Masson, 1979.

7. Ferreira SH. Prostaglandins, aspirin like drugs and analgesia. Nature New Biol 1972; **240**: 200.

8. Abelson MB, Chambers WA, Smith LW. Conjunctival allergen challenge: a clinical approach to studying allergic conjunctivitis. Acta Ophthalmol 1990; **108**: 84–8.

9. Abelson MB, Smith LM. Levocabastine. Evaluation in the histamine and compound 48/80 models of ocular allergy in humans. Ophthalmology 1988; **95**: 1494–7.

10. Abelson MB, Leonardi AA, Smith LM et al. Histaminase activity in patients with vernal keratoconjunctivitis. Ophthalmology 1995; **102**:1958–63.

11. Berdy GJ, Levene RB, Bateman ST et al. Identification of histaminase activity in human tears after conjunctival allergen challenge. Invest Ophthalmol Vis Sci 1990; **31**: 65.

12. Bonini S, Bonini S, Bucci MG et al. Allergen dose response and late symptoms in a human model of ocular allergy. J Allergy Clin Immunol 1990; **86**: 869–76.

13. Cipriandi G, Buscaglia S, Pesce G et al. Allergic subjects express intercellular adhesion molecule-1 (ICAM-1 or CD54) on epithelial cells of conjunctiva after allergen challenge. J Allergy Clin Immunol 1993; **91**: 783–92.

14. Schein OD, Munoz B, Tielsch JM et al. Prevalence of dry eye among the elderly. Am J Ophthalmol 1997; **124**: 723–8.

15. Doughty MJ, Fonn D, Richter D et al. A patient questionnaire approach to estimating the prevalence of dry eye symptoms in patients presenting to optometric practices across Canada. Optom Vis Sci 1997; **74**: 624–31.

16. Physicians' desk reference for ophthalmic medications. 30th Edn. Montvale: Medical Economics Company Inc., 2002.

17. Secchi A, Leonardi A, Discepola M et al. An efficacy and tolerance comparison of emedastine difumerate 0.05% and levocabastine hydrochloride 0.05%: reducing chemosis and eyelid swelling in subjects with seasonal allergic conjunctivitis. Emadine Study group. Acta Ophthalmol Scand Suppl 2000; **(230)**: 48–51.

18. Foster CS. Immunologic disorders of the conjunctiva, cornea and sclera. In: Principles and practices of ophthalmology: clinical practice. Albert DM, Jakobiec FA eds. Philadelphia: W B Saunders, 1994; p191.

19. Santos CI, Huang AJ, Abelson MB et al. Efficacy of lodoxamide 0.1% ophthalmic solution in resolving corneal epitheliopathy associated with vernal keratoconjunctivitis. Am J Ophthalmol 1994; **117(4)**: 488–97.

20. DeWeck AL, Derer T, Bahre M. Investigation of the anti-allergic activity of azelastine on the immediate and late-phase reactions to allergens and histamine using telethermography. Clin Exp Allergy 2000; **30**: 283–7.

21. Greiner JV, Michaelson C, McWhirter CL, Shams NB. Single dose of ketotifen fumarate 0.025% vs 2 weeks of cromolyn sodium 4% for allergic conjunctivitis. Adv Ther 2002; **19**: 185–93.

22. Aguilar AJ. Comparative study of clinical efficacy and tolerance in seasonal allergic conjunctivitis management with 0.1% olopatadine hydrochloride versus 0.05% ketotifen fumarate. Acta Ophthalmol Scand Suppl 2000; **(230)**: 52–5.

23. Welch DL, Ousler GO, Abelson MB. Ocular drying associated with oral antihistamines (Loratadine) in the normal population. Cornea 2000; **19**: S135.

24. Sharif NA, Xu SX, Miller ST et al. Characterization of the ocular antiallergic and antihistaminic effects of olopatadine (AL-4943A), a novel drug for treating ocular allergic diseases. JPET 1995; **278**: 1252–61.

25. Cook EB, Stahl JL, Barney NP, Graziano FM. Olopatadine inhibits TNF-alpha release from human conjunctival mast cells. Ann Allergy Asthma Immunol 2000; **84**: 504–8.

26. Cook EB, Stahl JL, Barney NP, Graziano FM. Olopatadine inhibits anti-immunoglobulin E-stimulated conjunctival mast cell upregulation of ICAM-1 expression on conjunctival epithelial cells. Ann Allergy Asthma Immunol 2001; **87**: 424–9.

27. Leonardi A, Abelson MB. Mast cell stabilizing effects of olopatadine following allergen challenge in humans. (Abstract) ARVO 2003.

28. Yanni JM, Stephens DJ, Miller ST et al. The in vitro and in vivo ocular pharmacology of olopatadine (AL-4943A): an effective anti-allergic/antihistaminic agent. J Ocul Pharmacol Ther 1996; **12**: 389–400.

29. Irkec M. Topical olopatadine decreases tear eotaxin in patients with seasonal allergic conjunctivitis (SAC). ARVO abstract # 3092.

30. Abelson MB, Turner FD, Amin D. Patanol is effective in the treatment of the signs and symptoms of allergic conjunctivitis and allergic rhinoconjunctivitis. Invest Ophthalmol Vis Sci 2000; **41(Suppl)**: 4922.

31. Butrus S, Geiner JV, Discepola M, Finegold I. Comparison of the clinical efficacy and comfort of olopatadine hydrochloride 0.1% ophthalmic solution and nedocromil sodium 2% ophthalmic solution in the human conjunctival allergen challenge model. Clin Ther 2000; **22**: 1462–72.

32. Berdy GJ, Spangler DL, Bensch G et al. A comparison of the relative efficacy and clinical performance of olopatadine hydrochloride 0.1% ophthalmic solution and ketotifen fumarate 0.025% ophthalmic solution in the conjunctival allergen challenge model. Clin Ther 2000; **22**: 826–33.

33. Spangler DL, Bensch G, Berdy GJ. Evaluation of the efficacy of olopatadine hydrochloride 0.1% ophthalmic solution and azelastine hydrochloride 0.05% ophthalmic solution in the conjunctival allergen challenge model. Clin Ther 2001; **23**: 1272–80.

34. D'Arienzo PA, Granet DB. Variability of drop comfort and its importance as a criterion in the selection of topical therapy for ocular allergy. AAAAI 2001.

35. Berdy GJ, Stoppel JO, Epstein AB. Comparison of the clinical efficacy and tolerability of olopatadine hydrochloride 0.1% ophthalmic solution and loteprednol etabonate 0.2% ophthalmic suspension in the conjunctival allergen challenge model. Clin Ther 2002; **24**: 918–29.

36. Abelson MB, Welch DL. An evaluation of onset and duration of action of Patanol (olopatadine hydrochloride ophthalmic solution 0.1%) compared to Claritin (loratadine 10 mg) tablets in acute allergic conjunctivitis in the conjunctival allergen challenge model. Acta Ophthalmol Scand Suppl 2000; **(230)**: 60–3.

37. Lanier BQ, Abelson MB, Berger WE et al. Comparison of the efficacy of combined fluticasone propionate and olopatadine versus combined fluticasone propionate and fexofenadine for the treatment of allergic rhinoconjunctivitis induced by conjunctival allergen challenge. Clin Ther 2002; **24**: 1161–74.

38. Brodsky M, Berger WE, Butrus S et al. Evaluation of comfort using olopatadine hydrochloride 0.1% ophthalmic solution in the treatment of allergic conjunctivitis in contact lens wearers compared to placebo using the conjunctival allergen challenge model. Eye and Contact Lens 2003; **29** (in press).

Discussion

MARTIN CHURCH: The ability of a human mast cell to respond to a drug does not depend on its chymase and tryptase. The uterine mast cells, for example, are like the skin's mast cells and the eye's mast cells. With nedocromil, the eye mast cells respond but the mast cells of the skin and uterus do not at all. Even if cells look the same, it does not mean that they will have the same response. Likewise, just because they look different, does not mean they respond differently: the skin mast cells have a complement receptor, but the eye's mast cells do not.

MARK ABELSON: You believe then that studies should be tissue- and species-specific. I think that is critical and that doctors should be aware of this when they evaluate the wealth of data available on new or historical agents. Pre-clinical data *in vivo* or *in vitro* must be tissue- and species-specific to allow extrapolation to the situation in humans. What we are really looking for is proof of clinical efficacy.

MARTIN CHURCH: One other point you must not overlook in research is that as soon as histamine is released, it causes vasodilatation, which facilitates washout by the bloodstream. With tests in the skin, drug concentrations drop as soon as vasodilatation occurs.

MARTIN CHURCH: You say that you have not seen evidence of a late phase in seasonal allergic conjunctivitis. Our study at the University of Southampton, UK, with the antigen challenge did show a late phase, with itching occurring late on [1]. I think that the response depends on the degree of challenge — certainly that is the case in every other organ that we have looked at. Unless the challenge is very strong, a late response will not be seen.

MARK ABELSON: You are correct that a late phase is only induced in a small subgroup that is challenged with high doses. I do not believe you can challenge patients more than we do without performing the challenge in the intensive care unit. To induce the late phase consistently would be dangerous for many patients as we see even with lower allergen challenges that patients get itching in the throat, which signifies that the mediators are draining into the throat — this could lead to respiratory problems if you are not careful.

DAVID EASTY: Has olopatadine been studied just in seasonal allergic conjunctivitis or has it been tried in vernal keratoconjunctivitis? Can it control symptoms of vernal conjunctivitis?

MARK ABELSON: There are studies by Aguilar and by Irkec [2].

DAVID EASTY: Vernal keratoconjunctivitis and atopic keratoconjunctivitis can be very difficult to treat, and until the second-generation mast cell stabilizers lodoxamide and nedocromil became available, we had to use steroids much more and thus had to deal with the concomitant problems. Now we are able to control these diseases more easily without using steroids — the side-effects are reduced, the patient's vision is better, and so on. If olopatadine can be proved to be superior to nedocromil, then it might help us reduce the need for steroids. For instance, it may prevent the acute exacerbations we see in vernal keratoconjunctivitis, by stopping the flare-up and stopping the corneal ulcers.

MARK ABELSON: We have that data very clearly for seasonal allergic conjunctivitis [3, 4]. In vernal keratoconjunctivitis we do not have comparative data for nedocromil, but such studies should be undertaken. I think initially that olopatadine will not be as good at suppressing the colony stimulating factors that increase the population of mast cells as steroids. I do believe, however, that it will allow the use of less steroid or will allow steroids to be tapered off more quickly than sodium cromoglycate and nedocromil.

References

1.   Bacon AS, Ahluwalia P, Irani AM et al. Tear and conjunctival changes during the allergen-induced early- and late-phase responses. J Allergy Clin Immunol 2000; **106**: 948–54.

2.   Irkec MT, Bozkurt B, Kerimoglu H et al. Tear cytokines in patients with vernal keratoconjunctivitis (VKC) responding clinically to topical olopatadine or additional rimexolone. ARVO (abstract) 2003.

3.   Leonardi A, Borghesan F, Faggian D et al. Eosinophil cationic protein in tears of normal subjects and patients affected by vernal keratoconjunctivitis. Allergy 1995; **50**: 610–13.

4.   Butrus S, Greiner JV, Discepola M, Finegold I. Comparison of the clinical efficacy and comfort of olopatadine hydrochloride 0.1% ophthalmic solution and nedocromil sodium 2% ophthalmic solution in the human conjunctival allergen challenge model. Clin Ther 2000; **22**: 1462–72.